# PEDIATRIC

## FOCUSED HISTORY TAKING AND CLINICAL EXAMINATION

HOT NOTES BY Dr. M.O.H.M.

# PEDIATRICS

## Contents:

**HISTORY TAKING**
  CASE SHEETs
  Jaundice $H_x$
  Hematuria
  Fit $H_x$
  Enuresis $H_x$
  Joint swelling $H_x$
  Diabetes mellitus $H_x$
  Diarrhea $H_x$
  Wheezy chest $H_x$
  Cough $H_x$
  Fever $H_x$
  Cardiac disease $H_x$

**EXAMINATION**
  General Ex
  Respiratory distress Assessment
  Hydration status assessment
  Nutritional status assessment
  Patient with meningitis
  Patient with bleeding tendency
  Patient with diabetes
  Patient with jaundice
  Patient with Hematuria
  Patient with diarrhea
  Patient with edema (N.S.)
  Patient with hydrocephalus
  Patient with rickets
  Down syndrome
  Temperature measurement
  Height measurement in children

**COMMUNICATION SKILLS**
  Diabetes mellitus ' Insulin injection '
  Diabetes mellitus ' Diabetes diet '
  Diabetes M. ' Hypoglycemic attacks '
  Diabetes M. ' How to use a glucometer '
  Lumbar puncture
  Breast feeding
  Oral rehydration solution (O.R.S.)
  Enuresis
  Vaccination
  Vaccines

**INVESTIGATIONS**
  Normal values
  Cerebrospinal fluid (C.S.F.) analysis
  N. S. vs. Glumerilunephritis
  Trick - Hematology

**FOLLOW UP CHARTS**

**DEVELOPMENT MADE VERY EASY**

**DRUGs ' ESSENTIAL NOTEs '**

**INTRAVENOUS FLUIDs**

**BLOOD PRODUCTs**

**OTHER IMPORTANT TOPICS**
  Lumbar puncture
  Bone marrow aspiration & biopsy
  Exchange transfusion
  Phototherapy
  Ventolin nubulizar (Salbutamol)
  Different types of drips
  Intraousseous needle
  Liver biopsy
  Urine analysis (Urine dipstick)
  Other important topics

# 5- PEDIATRICS     HISTORY TAKING [ CASE SHEET ]..

## HISTORY CASE SHEET :

### DEMOGRAPHY DATA:
Name:
Date of birth & age :
Sex :
Address :
Date of admission:
Date of taking history :
Source of history : *( patient, mother or both of them ? )*

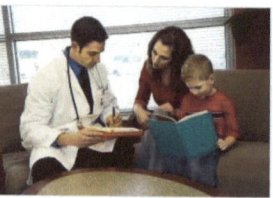

### CHIEF COMPLAINT & DURATION:

### H$_x$ OF PRESENT ILLNESS:

**Ask about :**

How and when the illness started ( SYSTEM INVOLVED ) ?

Any changes in the course of the illness ?

Any drugs are given ? any benefit ?

Mention the effect of illness on [ THE SIX ]:

Appetite ?

Weight ?

Bowel motion ?

Urine output ?

Sleep ?

Activity ?

Progress of illness in the hospital ?

### SYSTEMS REVIEW :

**Alimentary system & the abdomen:**

Difficulty in swallowing : For liquids or with solid food ?
                              Food stuck ? Level ?

Regurgitation : How often ?
                Aggravating factors ?
Heartburn ?
Vomiting : Any blood ?
Abdominal pain ? *( mention pain analysis )*
Abdominal distension ?

## 5- PEDIATRICS — HISTORY TAKING [ CASE SHEET ]..

Bowel motion : Diarrhea or constipation ?
Yellowish discoloration of sclera & skin ?
Diet : Type of food ? , Any food prevention ? , At what age did he start table food ?

**Respiratory system :**
Cough : In attacks ? , Whooping ?
Sputum ?
Nasal discharge ?
Shortness of breath :  At rest ? , At night ? , On exertion ?
　　　　　　　　　　Any previous attack ?
　　　　　　　　　　Associated symptoms : Cough ? , Increase body temperature ? ,
　　　　　　　　　　　　　　　　Bluish discoloration of the lips, face or limbs ?
　　　　　　　　　　Effect on feeding ?
　　　　　　　　　　Any family $H_x$ ?

Wheezing ?
Bluish discoloration of the lips, face or limbs ?
Chest pain : *( in appropriate age )*

**Cardiovascular system :**
Shortness of breath :  At rest ? , At night ? , On lying flat ? , Effect on feeding ?
Awareness of heart beats *( palpitation )* ?
Chest pain ?
Pallor ?
Bluish discoloration of the lips ,face ,limbs ?
Ankle swelling ?

**Genitourinary system :**
Urine stream ?
Any blood with urine ?
Loin pain ? *( mention pain analysis )*
Burning micturition ?
Testicular swelling ?
Puffy face, ankle swelling or abdominal distension ?
Shortness of breath ?

**Nervous system :**
Fits : Duration of complaint ?
　　　Date of 1st fit ? & Duration ?
　　　No. of fits /day ?
　　　What happen before & after it ?
　　　Child's condition between attacks ?
　　　Associated symptoms : Loss of consciousness ? , Tongue bite ?, Frothy secretion ?,
　　　　　　　　　　　Rolling of the eyes ? , Loss of sphincter control ? ,
　　　　　　　　　　　Verbalization ?

## 5- PEDIATRICS — HISTORY TAKING [ CASE SHEET ]..

Headache ?
Change in behavior ?
Change in activity ?
Change in gait or posture ?
Blurred vision ?

Chocking & cough with feeding ?

**Locomotor system :**
Limping ?
Limb swelling or pain ?
Bruises ?
Any deformity ?

### ANTENATAL $H_x$:

Maternal health before and during pregnancy ?
Attend antenatal care clinic regularly ?
$H_x$ of D.M. , Hypertension , Anemia or Bleeding ?
$H_x$ of infection *( TORCH)*, Fever , Rash , Cervical swellings ?
Any drug use ?
Smoking or Alcohol ?
$H_x$ of leaking liquor ?
Toxoid vaccine ?

### Natal $H_x$:

Normal vaginal bleeding or caesarian section ? Why ?
Difficulties & length of labor ?
Any analgesia was given ?
Any resuscitation ?
Cry immediately ? , Breath spontaneously ?
Pass meconium ?

Birth order ? , Birth weight ?
Gestational age ?

### Postnatal $H_x$:

Admission to ICU or delivered to mother ?
$H_x$ of jaundice , $H_x$ of photo-therapy , $H_x$ of blood exchange ?
Fit ?
Fever ?

## 5- PEDIATRICS — HISTORY TAKING [ CASE SHEET ]..

### PAST-MEDICAL Hx:
Any communicable disease : As Chickenpox , Mumps , Measles , Whooping cough or Chronic disease like D.M.
Previous hospitalization : in E.R. ?

### DRUG Hx:
Take any drugs ?
Allergy to drug ?
Allergy to food ?

### PAST-SURGICAL Hx:
Any previous operation ?
Anesthesia ?
Blood exchange ?

### FAMILY Hx:
FATHER & MOTHER → Age ? , Jobs ? , Health condition ? & Consanguinity ?
SIBLING → NO. ? , Age ? , Health condition ?
$H_x$ of Asthma , Eczema , Cardiovascular illness ... etc. ?
Any similar illness in the family ?
*$H_x$ of death* in the family ?

### SOCIO-ECONOMIC Hx:
Environment ( rural or urban ) ?
Water sanitation ?
Overcrowding in home ( No. of people in the room ) ?
Smokers in the home ?
Animal ( pets ) ?
Income of the family ?

### VACCINATION Hx:
Date & Site of vaccination ?
Check the schedule ( Vaccination program in Iraq ) ?
Sever reaction after vaccination ?
Date of last vaccine ?

## 5- PEDIATRICS — HISTORY TAKING [ CASE SHEET ]..

### FEEDING Hx:

Type : ( Breast , Bottle , mixed ) or solid food ?
    If bottle feeding → Why shift to bottle feeding ?
                            Frequency ?
                            Amount & duration ?
                            Good bottle sterilization ?
                            Date of introducing solid food ?

    If breast feeding → Frequency ?
                            Duration of feed ?
                          Any difficulties ?
                          Exclusive or not ?

### DEVELOPMENTAL Hx:

( Milestone ) ?? → *See page no. 176*

## 5- PEDIATRICS    focus HISTORY TAKING..

### Jaundice ' history taking ':

**FIRST:** greet the mother,
introduce yourself,

**START WITH DEMOGRAPHY:**

name, date of birth, sex, address,
date of admission & date of taking $H_x$, source of $H_x$..

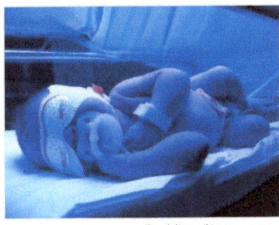

**CHIEF COMPLAINT & DURATION:**

**$H_x$ OF PRESENT ILLNESS:**

onset, at which day start ?, color of jaundice (lemon or green),

**urine & stool color**, **itching**, fever, convulsion, pallor or bleeding,

[ **weight, appetite, bowel motion, urine output, activity & sleep** ] = [ **THE 6** ]

↓↓ level of consciousness & fit (C.N.S.), abnormal behavior & school performance..

*then* complete the gastrointestinal system $H_x$ (frequent vomiting is very important)..

**PAST MEDICAL $H_x$:** bleeding, blindness or neuropathy (due to vit. K,E,D & A deficiency)..
**PAST SURGICAL $H_x$:**
**DRUG $H_x$: ASNANK** (**a**spirin, **s**ulfa drugs, **n**itrofurantoin, **a**nti-malarial, **n**alidixic acid, Vit.**K**) or depakin..

**FAMILY $H_x$:** mother & father blood group & Rh, similar condition, abortion or $H_x$ of death due to similar condition in the family..
**SOCIOECONOMIC $H_x$:** sanitation, pets..

**ANTENATAL CARE $H_x$:** take blood or plasma, had any fever or rash..
**NATAL $H_x$:** preterm ?, 1st child, normal vaginal delivery (N.V.D.) or by C/S..
**POST-NATAL $H_x$:** take exchange transfusion or photo$R_x$ ?, delay passage of meconium..

**VACCINATION $H_x$:** HBV vaccine ??
**FEEDING $H_x$:** bottle or breast, ingestion of fova beans..
**DEVELOPMENTAL $H_x$:** vision (head fixation & follow mother face), social smile ..etc

**& don't forget the REVIEW of SYSTEMS:**

At the end: thank the mother..

## 5- PEDIATRICS — focus HISTORY TAKING..

### Hematuria ' history taking ':

**FIRST:** greet the mother & the patient,
introduce yourself,

**START WITH DEMOGRAPHY:**
name, date of birth, sex, address,
date of admission & date of taking $H_x$, source of $H_x$..

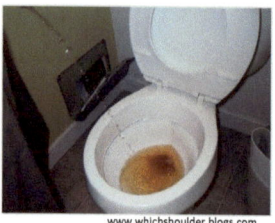

**CHIEF COMPLAINT, ONSET & DURATION:**

**$H_x$ OF PRESENT ILLNESS:**

skin infection before few weeks *or* upper respiratory tract infection before few days..,

frequency, urgency or painful micturition..

amount & color of urine,

body swelling, abdominal or flank pain, fever or rash,

bleeding, hemoptysis, stool color, trauma or heavy exercise..

loss of consciousness (encephalopathy) or headache,

[ **weight, appetite, bowel motion, urine output, activity & sleep** ] = [ **THE 6** ]

**PAST MEDICAL $H_x$:** photosensitivity ?
**PAST SURGICAL $H_x$:**
**DRUG $H_x$:**

**FAMILY $H_x$:** sickle cell disease..
**SOCIOECONOMIC $H_x$:**

**ANTENATAL CARE $H_x$:**
**NATAL $H_x$:**
**POST-NATAL $H_x$:**

*Trick:* Don't forget the $H_x$ must be in the patient words..
So, instead of Hematuria → we say red color urine
& so on.. [ this is a general *important* note.. ]

**VACCINATION $H_x$:**
**FEEDING $H_x$:**
**DEVELOPMENTAL $H_x$:**

& don't forget the REVIEW of SYSTEMS: ' if > 12 y. old → the *menstrual $H_x$* is very important '

At the end: thank the mother..

# 5- PEDIATRICS    focus HISTORY TAKING..

## Fit ' history taking ':

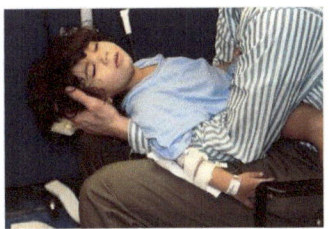

**FIRST:** greet the mother,
introduce yourself,

**START WITH DEMOGRAPHY:**
name, date of birth, sex, address,
date of admission & date of taking $H_x$, source of $H_x$..

**CHIEF COMPLAINT & DURATION:**

**$H_x$ OF PRESENT ILLNESS:**

onset, frequency, time of first fit ?, *What happen before the fit* ?

*describe the attack* → generalized, focal, tonic, or clonic, abnormal eye movements,
drooling of saliva, verbalization, tongue bite, bluish
discoloration, blurred vesion, incontinence or abnormal behavior..

trauma, diarrhea, fever or loss of consciousness, any aggravated factors..

*what happen after attack* ?, how to stop the attack?,

[ **weight, appetite, bowel motion, urine output, activity & sleep** ] = [ **THE 6** ]

*then* complete the C.N.S. system $H_x$

**PAST MEDICAL $H_x$:**
**PAST SURGICAL $H_x$:**
**DRUG $H_x$:**

**FAMILY $H_x$:** similar condition in the family ?
**SOCIOECONOMIC $H_x$:**

**ANTENATAL CARE $H_x$:** D.M. or T.O.R.C.H..
**NATAL $H_x$:** any complication, preterm, delay crying & meconium aspiration..
**POST-NATAL $H_x$:** jaundice..

**VACCINATION $H_x$:** pertusis, MMR..
**FEEDING $H_x$:**
**DEVELOPMENTAL $H_x$:** (IMPORTANT..)

**& don't forget the REVIEW of SYSTEMS:** it is very important especially the respiratory &
cardiovascular systems

**At the end:** thank the mother..

# 5- PEDIATRICS — focus HISTORY TAKING..

## Enuresis ' history taking ':

**FIRST:** greet the mother & the patient,
introduce yourself,

### START WITH DEMOGRAPHY:
name, date of birth, sex, address,
date of admission & date of taking $H_x$, source of $H_x$..

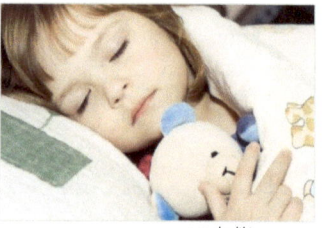

### CHIEF COMPLAINT & DURATION:

### $H_x$ OF PRESENT ILLNESS:

previously toilet trained or never attained control ? ($1°$ or $2°$ ?)

frequency (how many time per day & per week), at daytime or at night ?,

sleep after that ?

ask about the urine & complete the urinary system (in day time)..

fluid intake, emotional stress (family problems..etc)

**[ THE 6 ]..**

**PAST MEDICAL $H_x$:** D.M., mental retarded, U.T.I or any renal abnormality..
**PAST SURGICAL $H_x$:**
**DRUG $H_x$:**

**FAMILY $H_x$:** similar condition in the family ?
**SOCIOECONOMIC $H_x$:**

**ANTENATAL CARE $H_x$:**
**NATAL $H_x$:**
**POST-NATAL $H_x$:**

**VACCINATION $H_x$:**
**FEEDING $H_x$:**
**DEVELOPMENTAL $H_x$:**

**& don't forget the REVIEW of SYSTEMS:**

At the end: thank the mother..

# 5- PEDIATRICS     focus HISTORY TAKING..

## Bleeding tendency ' history taking ':

**FIRST:** greet the mother & the patient,
introduce yourself,

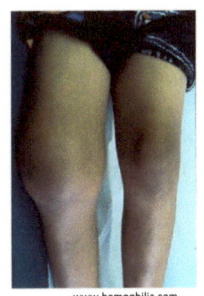
www.hemophilia.com

**START WITH DEMOGRAPHY:**
name, date of birth, sex, address,
date of admission & date of taking $H_x$, source of $H_x$..

**CHIEF COMPLAINT & DURATION:**

**$H_x$ OF PRESENT ILLNESS:**

site → skin , mucous mm, deep joints & mm. , GIT , urine color

severity, spontaneous or after trauma ?, correlation with the degree of injury

pallor, fever, bone pain , joint swelling

other autoimmune disease?

Type of bleeding → patechae, echymmosis, hematoma & their sites, no. , shape & color..

Jaundice? or headache , blurred vision (intracranial hemorrhage)

[ **THE 6** ]..

**PAST MEDICAL $H_x$:** previous attack, any $I_x$ (BT, PT, PTT, CBC, platelets function test, TT, clotting factors, mixing study)..

**PAST SURGICAL $H_x$:** tonsillectomy, circumcision, dental procedure? & take plasma ,cryo or platelets ?

**DRUG $H_x$:** aspirin or wrfarin

**FAMILY $H_x$:** similar condition in the family
**SOCIOECONOMIC $H_x$:**

*Trick: In joint swelling Hx. ask the following questions :*
*onset, which joints ?, no. of joints ?, is this the 1st attack ?,*
*fever, rash or weight loss & night sweating,*
*swelling or redness, early morning stiffness.*
*trauma.   mouth ulcer & red eye..*
*pain & bleeding tendency Hx.*
*[ the 6 ].*

**ANTENATAL CARE $H_x$:**
**NATAL $H_x$:**
**POST-NATAL $H_x$:**

**VACCINATION $H_x$:** any bleeding or swelling at the site of vaccination..
**FEEDING $H_x$:**
**DEVELOPMENTAL $H_x$:**

**& don't forget the REVIEW of SYSTEMS:**

At the end: thank you..

## 5- PEDIATRICS — focus HISTORY TAKING..

### Diabetes mellitus ' history taking ':

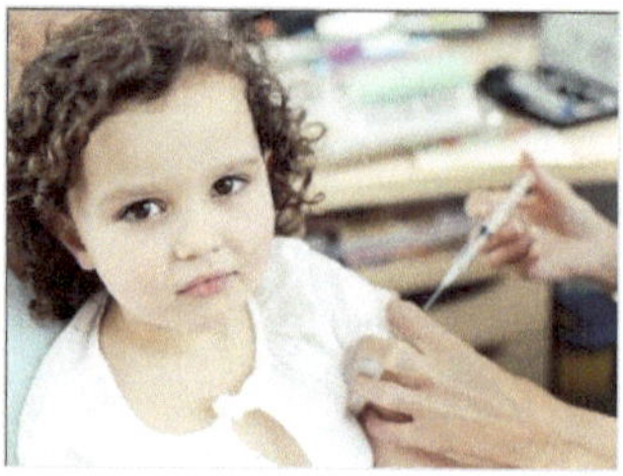

**FIRST:** greet the mother & the patient,
introduce yourself,

**START WITH DEMOGRAPHY:**
name, date of birth, sex, address,
date of admission & date of taking $H_x$, source of $H_x$..

**CHIEF COMPLAINT & DURATION:**

**$H_x$ OF PRESENT ILLNESS:**

onset, polyuria, nocturia, polydipsia, hyperphagia & weight loss,

for D.K.A → *disturbed level of consciousness*, *abdominal discomfort*, nausea & *vomiting*, dehydration, weakness or *deep heavy rapid respiration*..

↓↓ mentality ??

*trauma.. stress ?* or hypoglycemic attack or enuresis..

in ♀ *patient* → any abnormal discharge or itching..

[ **THE 6** ]..

**PAST MEDICAL $H_x$:** celiac disease, vitiligo, thyroid or S.L.E.
**PAST SURGICAL $H_x$:**
**DRUG $H_x$:** (IMPORTANT..)

**FAMILY $H_x$:** celiac disease..
**SOCIOECONOMIC $H_x$:** psychological stress..

**ANTENATAL CARE $H_x$:** rubella or maternal D.M.
**NATAL $H_x$:**
**POST-NATAL $H_x$:**

**VACCINATION $H_x$:**
**FEEDING $H_x$:**
**DEVELOPMENTAL $H_x$:**

*Trick: Don't forget the $H_x$ must be in the patient words.. So, instead of hyperphagia → we say increased consumption of food & so on.. [ this is a general important note.. ]*

**& don't forget the REVIEW of SYSTEMS:**

At the end: thank the mother..

## 5- PEDIATRICS — focus HISTORY TAKING..

### Diarrhea ' history taking ':

FIRST: greet the mother & the patient,
introduce yourself,

START WITH DEMOGRAPHY:
name, date of birth, sex, address,
date of admission & date of taking $H_x$, source of $H_x$..

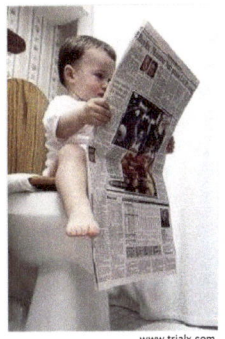

CHIEF COMPLAINT & DURATION:

$H_x$ OF PRESENT ILLNESS:

onset, amount, frequency, consistency & odor,

color, mucus or blood..

fever, abdominal pain or distension, vomiting or tensmus

related to feeding

*then* complete the gastrointestinal system $H_x$..

[ **THE 6** ]..

PAST MEDICAL $H_x$:
PAST SURGICAL $H_x$:
DRUG $H_x$: (IMPORTANT..)

FAMILY $H_x$: similar condition in the family ?
SOCIOECONOMIC $H_x$: water supply & sanitation..

ANTENATAL CARE $H_x$:
NATAL $H_x$:
POST-NATAL $H_x$:

VACCINATION $H_x$:
FEEDING $H_x$: bottle or breast feeding ?
DEVELOPMENTAL $H_x$:

& don't forget the REVIEW of SYSTEMS:

At the end: thank the mother..

## 5- PEDIATRICS  focus HISTORY TAKING..

### Wheezy chest ' history taking ':

Trick: ' PEASE, SEE THE NEXT PAGE. '

FIRST:  greet the mother & the patient,
           introduce yourself,

START WITH DEMOGRAPHY:
   name, date of birth, sex, address,
   date of admission & date of taking $H_x$, source of $H_x$..

CHIEF COMPLAINT & DURATION:

$H_x$ OF PRESENT ILLNESS:

   onset, increased at specific time ?,

   cough (*especially after crying or at night*) or blush discoloration of the face & lips,

   fever or vomiting..

   foreign body aspiration ??

   *then* complete the respiratory system $H_x$..

   [ THE 6 ]..

PAST MEDICAL $H_x$: eczema, any previous hospitalization ?
PAST SURGICAL $H_x$:
DRUG $H_x$:

FAMILY $H_x$: asthma, cystic fibrosis, immunodeficiency or similar condition in the family ?
SOCIOECONOMIC $H_x$: smokers at home ?, pet ?..  overcrowding  ?

ANTENATAL CARE $H_x$:
NATAL $H_x$: gestational age ?, any intubation ?
POST-NATAL $H_x$:

VACCINATION $H_x$: (IMPORTANT..)
FEEDING $H_x$: any feeding difficulty ?, any new food exposure ?
DEVELOPMENTAL $H_x$:

& don't forget the REVIEW of SYSTEMS:

At the end: thank the mother..

# 5- PEDIATRICS    focus HISTORY TAKING..

## Cough ' history taking ':

Trick: ' PLEASE, SEE THE PREVIOUS PAGE. '

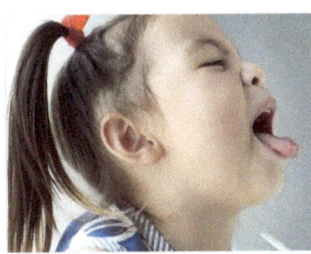

FIRST:  greet the mother & the patient,
introduce yourself,

START WITH DEMOGRAPHY:
name, date of birth, sex, address,
date of admission & date of taking $H_x$, source of $H_x$..

CHIEF COMPLAINT & DURATION:

$H_x$ OF PRESENT ILLNESS:

productive or not ?

frequency, continuous or intermitted ?, any diurnal variation ?

character ?..

any → chest pain, wheeze, bluish discoloration, change in the level of consciousness,
fever or vomiting..

weight loss & sweating → [ THE 6 ]..

PAST MEDICAL $H_x$:
PAST SURGICAL $H_x$:
DRUG $H_x$:

FAMILY $H_x$: similar condition in the family ?
SOCIOECONOMIC $H_x$: (IMPORTANT..)

ANTENATAL CARE $H_x$:
NATAL $H_x$:
POST-NATAL $H_x$:

VACCINATION $H_x$:
FEEDING $H_x$:
DEVELOPMENTAL $H_x$:

& don't forget the REVIEW of SYSTEMS:

At the end: thank the mother..

# 5- PEDIATRICS — focus HISTORY TAKING..

## Fever ' history taking ':

**FIRST:** greet the mother,
introduce yourself,

**START WITH DEMOGRAPHY:**
name, date of birth, sex, address,
date of admission & date of taking $H_x$, source of $H_x$..

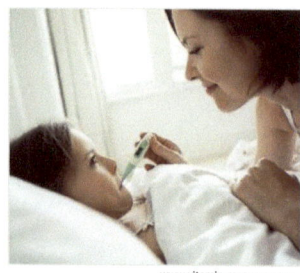

**CHIEF COMPLAINT & DURATION:**

**$H_x$ OF PRESENT ILLNESS:**

continuous, intermitted or remitted, severity, sweating & shivering,

at specific time.. nausea or projectile..

relieving factors → drugs, antipyretic or cold sponge

associated symptoms → convulsion, blush discoloration of the face & lips, headache,
weight loss, rash, jaundice,
joint pain, swelling, warmth or stiffness..

[ **THE 6** ]..

**PAST MEDICAL $H_x$:**
**PAST SURGICAL $H_x$:**
**DRUG $H_x$:**

**FAMILY $H_x$:**
**SOCIOECONOMIC $H_x$:**

**ANTENATAL CARE $H_x$:** (IMPORTANT.. → fever, rash, ....... sexual transmitted disease)
**NATAL $H_x$:** (IMPORTANT.. → premature, prolonged rupture membrane & chorioamnionitis )
**POST-NATAL $H_x$:**

**VACCINATION $H_x$:**
**FEEDING $H_x$:**
**DEVELOPMENTAL $H_x$:**

**& don't forget the REVIEW of SYSTEMS:** (IMPORTANT..)
(The important causes → U.T.I., meningitis, dysentery, joint & bone infection, sepsis)

At the end: thank the mother..

## 5- PEDIATRICS    focus HISTORY TAKING..

### Cardiac diseases ' history taking ':

FIRST: greet the mother,
introduce yourself,

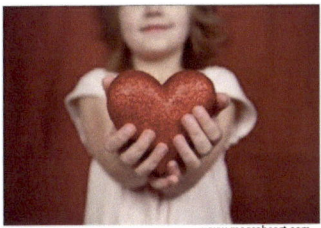

START WITH DEMOGRAPHY:
name, date of birth, sex, address,
date of admission & date of taking $H_x$, source of $H_x$..

CHIEF COMPLAINT & DURATION:

$H_x$ OF PRESENT ILLNESS:

shortness of breath (during feeding, at night or when lying flat),

chest pain,

bluish discoloration of the face & lips,

fatigue or leg swelling,

failure to thrive → [ **THE 6** ]..

PAST MEDICAL $H_x$:
PAST SURGICAL $H_x$:
DRUG $H_x$:

FAMILY $H_x$: heart problems or similar condition in the family ?
SOCIOECONOMIC $H_x$:

ANTENATAL CARE $H_x$: gestational D.M., medication, S.L.E., substance abuse or maternal rubella..
NATAL $H_x$: premature, bluish discoloration of the face & lips or respiratory distress..
POST-NATAL $H_x$:

VACCINATION $H_x$:
FEEDING $H_x$: any difficulty ?, frequency..
DEVELOPMENTAL $H_x$:

& don't forget the REVIEW of SYSTEMS:

At the end: thank the mother..

# 5- PEDIATRICS — EXAMINATION..

## General examination:

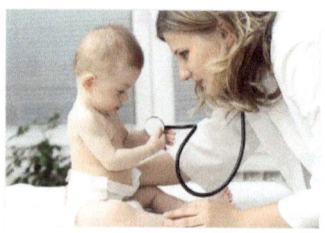

**First:** greet the patient & the mother,
introduce yourself,
take permission for examination,
*hand washing,*
make sure patient privacy,
good exposure *' when needed..'*

**General look:** *' for example '*, a ♀ infant, lying flat in the bed,
she look well, comfortable, conscious, alert, oriented *(for place, person and time),*
not dyspneic, no wheeze & no stridor,
no dysmprphic features & no specific complexion,
with yellow i.v. cannula in her right hand, no i.v. fluid, no $O_2$ bottle ….etc

**Head:** anterior fontanelle (*sitting & quite*),
eye → jaundice, pallor, tear, conjunctival hemorrhage, pre-orbital edema & malar rash,
ear → low set ears ?
nose → nasal flaring,
lips & mouth → cyanosis, jaundice, pallor, angular stomatitis, moist ?, thrush,
gum (any bleeding ?), tongue, tonsils & palate..

**Neck:** L.N. & thyroid gland..

**Hand:** pallor, cyanosis, clubbing, edema, splinter hemorrhage, hot & sweating,
palmer erythema, koilonychias, any deformity or Osler's nodes..

**Arm & forearm:** radial pulse (*vital signs*) & skin lesions (rash, bruises, hematoma, petechiae,
vitiligo & café au lait),

**Axilla:** L.N.

**Chest:** inspection → deformity, movement ..etc, [ **signs of respiratory distress** ]..

**Abdomen:** distention..etc, skin turgor [ **nutritional assessment** ]..

**Lower limb & Genitalia:** edema, skin lesion, joint swelling, deformity, inguinal L.N.,
, genitalia & napkin area → *dermatitis, stool & ambiguous genitalia..*

**Don't forget:** [ *Nutritional assessment* ], [ *Dehydration assessment* ], [ *Growth parameters* ]..

**At the end:** cover the patient & thank the mother..  *Trick: This is an important step in the all next topics..*

## 5- PEDIATRICS — EXAMINATION..

### Respiratory distress assessment:

First: greet the patient & the mother,
introduce yourself,
take permission for examination,
*hand washing,*
make sure patient privacy,
good exposure *' when needed..'*

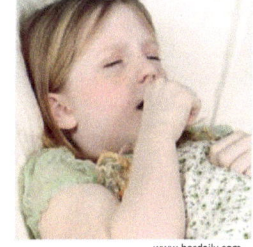

Then examine: consciousness,
wheeze, grunting, stridor,

alar nose flaring,
cyanosis,

retraction (suprasternal, intercostals & subcostal),
use of accessory muscles,

vital signs (respiratory rate..),
complete chest examination..

At the end: cover the patient & thank the mother..

---

### Hydration status assessment:

First: greet the patient & the mother,
introduce yourself,
take permission for examination,
*hand washing,*
make sure patient privacy,
good exposure *' when needed..'*

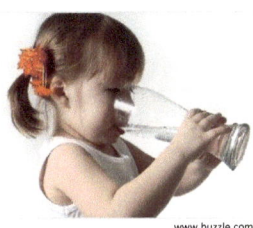

Then examine: *consciousness,*
*eager to drink,*
*skin turgor,*

fontanelle (depressed ?),
eye (sunken ?, tears ?),
mouth (dry ?),

capillary refilling (press on the sternum 5 sec.),

urine output,

vital signs & growth parameters..

At the end: cover the patient & thank the mother..

# 5- PEDIATRICS — EXAMINATION..

### Nutritional status assessment:

First: greet the patient & the mother,
introduce yourself,
take permission for examination,
*hand washing,*
make sure patient privacy,
good exposure *' when needed..'*

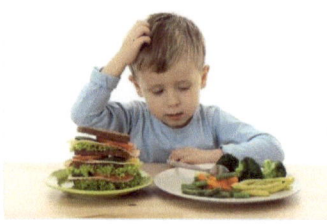
www.childrenssite.net

General look: **apathy** (kwashiorkor) or **irritable** (marasmus),

Signs of wasting: buttock,
inner thigh,
mid-upper arm circumference,
master muscles,

Edema:

Skin: wrinkling, pealing or darkening,

Mouth: angular stomatitis, tongue atrophy,

Growth parameters: OFC, weight, height,

Other: hair → flag sign in kwashiorkor, easily removed in marasmus..
orifices → acrodermatitis enteropathica..
signs of rickets or iron deficiency anemia..
liver enlargement..
abdominal distension..

At the end: cover the patient & thank the mother..

---

★★ For **cardiovascular system**, respiratory, nervous, G.I.T. systems examination, you can see chapter *' 1 '..* (with some differences because the child may be not compliant in some steps)..

## 5- PEDIATRICS — EXAMINATION..

### Patient with meningitis:

First: greet the patient & the mother,
introduce yourself,
take permission for examination,
*hand washing,*
make sure patient privacy,
good exposure *' when needed..'*

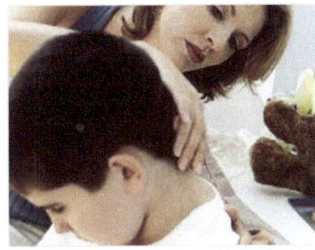

General: consciousness, posture & skin,

Vital signs:

Meningeal signs:

Fontanelle & OFC + Pupil & fundoscopy:

Neuro-examination: cranial nerves,
upper & lower limbs,

Then: complete the growth parameters..

At the end: cover the patient & thank him..

## 5- PEDIATRICS — EXAMINATION..

### Patient with bleeding tendency (or pallor):

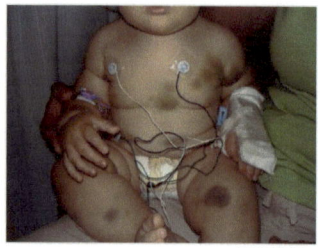

First: greet the patient & the mother,
introduce yourself,
take permission for examination,
*hand washing,*
make sure patient privacy,
good exposure *' when needed..'*

General look:

Head: pallor & jaundice,
L.N.
subconjunctival hemorrhage, gum bleeding, tongue, lips, fontanelle & fundoscopy,

Neck: L.N.

Hand: pallor, nail-bed, cyanosis, clubbing,
palmer erythema, koilonychias,
cannula site,

Arm & forearm: radial pulse (*vital signs*),
skin lesions (rash ' *fade with pressure* ', bruises, hematoma or petechiae),

Axilla: L.N.

Chest: spider nevi & heart auscultation,

Abdomen: especially for hepatosplenomegaly,

Legs: edema & ***joints swelling***,

Neurological examination: especially the reflexes (Babinski)..

You can see: the urine & stool color, if there is any sample..

At the end: cover the patient & thank the mother..

## 5- PEDIATRICS — EXAMINATION..

### Patient with diabetes:

First: greet the patient & the mother,
introduce yourself,
take permission for examination,
*hand washing,*
make sure patient privacy,
good exposure *'when needed..'*

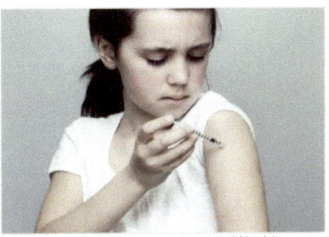

General look: consciousness, hydration status & any dysmorphic features,

Growth parameters: weight & height,

Vital signs: respiratory rate, radial pulse & blood pressure & temperature,

Abdomen: distension.

Site of injection: lypohypertrophy,
Site of infection: interdigital spaces or vaginal infection,

Prayer sign:

Skin (vitiligo), thyroid & eye (cataract):

Look for any other complication..

At the end: cover the patient & thank the mother..

## 5- PEDIATRICS — EXAMINATION..

**Patient with jaundice:**

First: greet the patient & the mother,
introduce yourself,
take permission for examination,
*hand washing,*
make sure patient privacy,
good exposure *' when needed..'*

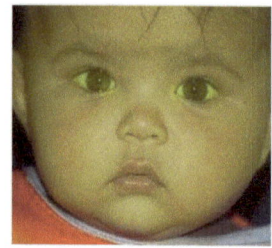
www.dailyhealthreport.com

General look: consciousness & dysmorphic features,

Head: jaundice & pallor,
Scalp for hematoma, cataract,

Neck: L.N.

Hand: pallor, nail bed, clubbing, palmer erythema & cyanosis,

Arm & forearm: radial pulse (*vital signs*),
skin lesions (rash ' *fade with pressure* ', bruises, hematoma or petechiae),

Axilla: L.N.,

Chest: spider nevi,

Abdomen: compete examination.. (*especially for hepatosplenomegaly* & umbilical hernia),

Legs: edema,

Napkin area: for stool & urine color..

You can see: the urine & stool color, if there is any sample..

Don't forget: *[ Nutritional assessment ], [ Dehydration assessment ], [ Growth parameters ],*
*[ primitive reflex (moro reflex) ]..*

At the end: cover the patient & thank the mother..

## 5- PEDIATRICS — EXAMINATION..

### Patient with hematuria:

First: greet the patient & the mother,
introduce yourself,
take permission for examination,
*hand washing,*
make sure patient privacy,
good exposure *'when needed..'*

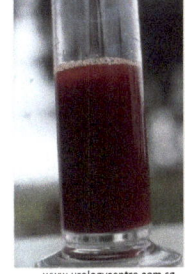

General look:

Head: tonsils, malar rash & periorbital edema,

Hand:
Arm & forearm: radial pulse & B.P. (*vital signs*),
skin lesions (rash '*fade with pressure*', bruises, hematoma or petechiae),

Abdomen: renal mass & renal angle tenderness,

Genitalia: infection or truma

At the end: cover the patient & thank the mother..

---

### Patient with diarrhea:

First: greet the patient & the mother,
introduce yourself,
take permission for examination,
*hand washing,*
make sure patient privacy,
good exposure *'when needed..'*

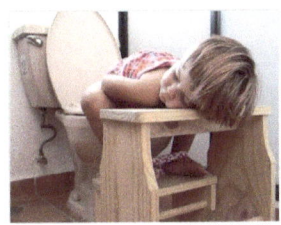

General look:
Dehydration status:
Nutritional status:
Growth parameters:

Vital signs:
Look for any signs of infection: (*otitis media, tonsillitis, U.T.I or viral..*)
Napkin area:

At the end: cover the patient & thank the mother..

## 5- PEDIATRICS — EXAMINATION..

### Patient with edema (Nephrotic syndrome):

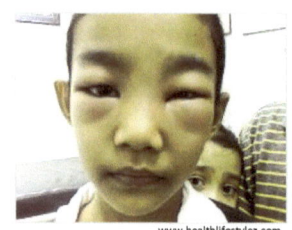

First: greet the patient & the mother,
introduce yourself,
take permission for examination,
***hand washing,***
make sure patient privacy,
good exposure *' when needed..'*

General look: periorbital puffiness,
leg edema,
abdominal distension,

Leg: edema,
pigmintation (*to differentiate between Kwashorkor & Nephrotic syndrome*),

Abdomen: ascitis (*shifting dullness & transmitted thrill*)

Chest: plural effusion,

Trick: Whenever you want to *touch the patient*, you have to ask him if he has any pain & you have to look to his face ' to observe his facial expression '..

Arm & forearm: swelling,

Genitalia: swelling,

### Side effect of steroid:

Vital signs:

Don't forget: [ *Nutritional assessment* ],
[ *Growth parameters* ],

Trick: Steroid S.E. ' CUSHING MAP ':..
C → cataract, cushing's syndrome (iatrogenic)
U → peptic ulcer
S → stria
H → hirsutism, hyperglycemia, hypertension
I → infection, ↓↓ immunity, insomnia
N → necrosis of femoral head (avascular necrosis)
G → growth retardation
S → psychosis
M → myopathy (proximal type)
A → acne, acute adrenal failure (after sudden withdrawal)
P → porosis (osteo-), pancreatitis

At the end: cover the patient & thank the mother..

## 5- PEDIATRICS   EXAMINATION..

### Patient with hydrocephalus:

First: greet the patient & the mother,
introduce yourself,
take permission for examination,
*hand washing,*
make sure patient privacy,
good exposure *' when needed..'*

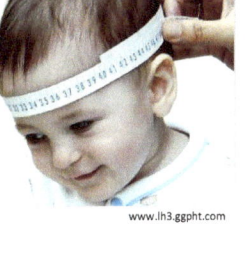

General look:

*OFC:* take 3 measures & consider the largest number.
*Fontanelle & sun set eyes:*
*Sutures & dilated veins:*
*Transillumination:*
*Cracked pot sign:* when you tap on the skull → abnormal sound..

for ↑↑ I.C.P.: examine the (vital signs, papilledema & cranial nerves),
Ventriculoperitoneal shunt: examine the course of the shunt..

At the end: cover the patient & thank the mother..

---

### Patient with rickets:

First: greet the patient & the mother,
introduce yourself,
take permission for examination,
*hand washing,*
make sure patient privacy,
good exposure *' when needed..'*

General look:

*Wide fontanelle:*
*Craniotabes:* (The bone is soft and when pressure is applied they will collapse underneath it. When the pressure is relieved, the bones will usually snap back into place).
*Bossing:*
*Teeth:*

*Rachitic rosary:*
*Harrison's sulcus:* (*subcostal*)

*Widening of radial & ulnar ends:*
*Bow legs & delayed walking:*
*Abdominal examination:*

At the end: cover the patient & thank the mother..

## 5- PEDIATRICS — EXAMINATION..

### Down syndrome (trisomy 21):

First: greet the patient & the mother,
introduce yourself,
take permission for examination,
*hand washing,*
make sure patient privacy,
good exposure '*when needed..*'

General look:

Head: flat occiput,
flat facial profile,
excess nuchal skin,
fontanelle,
slanted palpebral fissure, epicanthal fold, brushfield spot in eyes,
low set ears,
small jaw,

Hand: single crease (*simian crease*), short thick fingers & $5^{th}$ finger dysplasia,

Legs: flat achillis tendon & crease between the $1^{st}$ & $2^{nd}$ toes (apes' groove)..

Nervous system examination: hypotonia, frog like posture & poor neonatal reflexes,

Chest: heart auscultation,

Abdominal examination:

At the end: cover the patient & thank the mother..

www.independentspeech.files.wordpress.com

### Temperature measurement:

The mercury thermometer degrees: 35 - 42 °C

Routs: Oral,
Axillary corrected (+ 0.5° C) ' *Safest* ',
Rectally corrected (- 0.5° C),
Aural..

Normal body temperature is: 36.5 - 37.5 °C

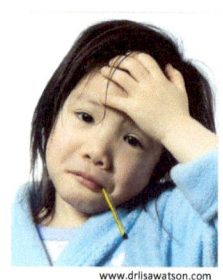

www.drlisawatson.com

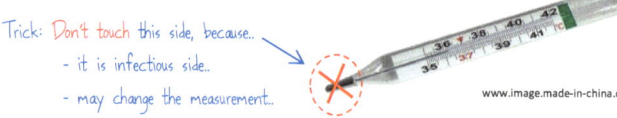

Trick: Don't touch this side, because..
- it is infectious side..
- may change the measurement..

www.image.made-in-china.com

## 5- PEDIATRICS — EXAMINATION..

### Height measurement in children:

**First:** greet the patient & the mother,

introduce yourself,

take permission for examination,

*hand washing,*

make sure patient privacy,

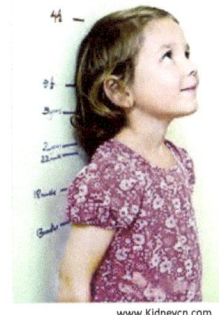

**Then:**
1. Remove the child's shoes, bulky clothing, and hair ornaments, and unbraid hair that interferes with the measurement.
2. Take the height measurement on flooring that is not carpeted and against a flat surface such as a wall with no molding.
3. Have the child stand with feet flat, together, and against the wall. Make sure legs are straight, arms are at sides, and shoulders are level.
4. Make sure the child is looking straight ahead and that the line of sight is parallel with the floor.
5. Take the measurement while the child stands with head, shoulders, buttocks, and heels touching the flat surface (wall). (See illustration.) Depending on the overall body shape of the child, all points may not touch the wall.
6. Use a flat headpiece to form a right angle with the wall and lower the headpiece until it firmly touches the crown of the head.
7. Make sure the measurer's eyes are at the same level as the headpiece.
8. Lightly mark where the bottom of the headpiece meets the wall. Then, use a metal tape to measure from the base on the floor to the marked measurement on the wall to get the height measurement.
9. Plot the result on the chart..

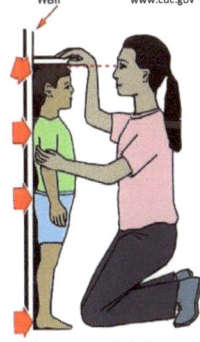

# 5- PEDIATRICS — COMMUNICATION SKILLS..

Trick: *'You have to use the country native language..'*

## Diabetes mellitus ' Insulin injection ':

### INSULIN INJECTION:

Greet the mother & introduce yourself,
Take permission..

There are *2 types* of syringes (even and odd )..
There are *3 types* of insulin (soluble, lente & mixed)..

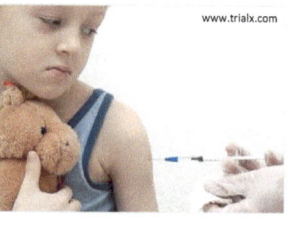

The even syringe:
   Each line equivalent to **two** units of insulin,
     (between no.0 and number 10 there are only **five** lines)..

The odd syringe:
   Each line equivalent to **one** units of insulin,
     (between no.0 and number 10 there are **ten** lines)..

*You have to draw up the **soluble** insulin before the insoluble..*

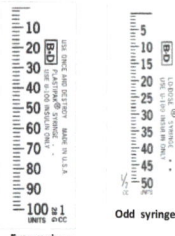

**Sites of injections** → outer arm, abdomen, outer thigh & hip area.. [ *subcutaneously* ]..

   *Injection is either by 45° or by a lifted skin fold method (lift the skin between thumb and two fingers with one hand, pulling the skin and fat away from the underlying muscle, and holding until the insulin has been injected )..*

The site *should be changed* at each injection (rotated) to reduce the risk of skin thickness (lipohypertrophy) developing. A simple way to reduce this risk is to systematically rotate the site where the insulin is injected..

**INSULIN:** There are **3 types** of insulin :

   Soluble (yellow vial, clear solution), lente (light blue or green vial, cloudy), mixed (brown, written on it *30 \ 70*)..

   You have to keep it in the refrigerator (but not in freeze), because it is a protein (damaged by heat)..

### DOSE CALCULATION: *' according to age & weight '*

*Weight* **X 0.7** = no. of insulin units (2/3 at the morning, 1/3 at evening ),
                         (1/3 soluble, 2/3 lente )..

*For example*, if the child's weight is *21.5* kg. → he need *21.5* **X 0.7** = 15 units of insulin..
                 (10 unit at the morning, 5 at evening ), (1/3 soluble, 2/3 lente)..

**You have to plot a chart** (date & time, blood sugar reading & insulin dose..)

**AT THE END:** thank the mother..

# 5- PEDIATRICS   COMMUNICATION SKILLS..

## Diabetes mellitus ' Diabetes diet ':

Trick: *'You have to use the country **native** language..'*

Greet the mother & introduce yourself,
Take permission..

Daily, 3 meals & 3 snacks..

Sugars (**55%**):
- Table sugar is forbidden..
- Potato, rice & breads → You have to choose one in each meal & reduce its amount..
- Fruits → one piece each day..

Fat (**30%**):
- Use vegetable oils only..

Proteins (**15%**):
- Use white meat only.. (*red meat is forbidden..*)

**Don't** provide all kinds of food in the refrigerator..

After each dose of insulin, the child **should eat**..

If the child *refuses to dine* (*for example*), he **should not** take the evening dose of insulin..

If the child *insists* to eat something (chocolate for example) → **he can**, *but either after* taking a dose of insulin **or** going to run or play football (*it is just an example*)..

Always, keep something sweet in the child's pocket..

**Thank the mother..**


## Diabetes mellitus ' hypoglycemic attacks ':

Greet the mother & introduce yourself,
Take permission..

You have to know hypoglycemic attack symptoms & how to deal with it..
- mild: *pallor, sweating, tearfulness, irritability & aggression..*
- moderate: *drowsy, confusion & personality changes..*
- sever symptoms: *inability to seek help & seizures or coma..*

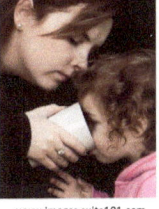

So, give him something sweet (*like an orange juice..*), then after 5 min, check the blood sugar [ *if it is of no benefit or he can't drink* → inject him with glucagon.. ]

*You have to plot a chart* (*date & time, blood sugar reading & insulin dose*)..

**Causes of hypoglycemia:** Changed the person, the syringe or insulin type..
Stress or sever exercise (*especially after the insulin dose*)..
There is a gap between the insulin dose and the meal..
Infection (hepatitis)..
Nephropathy..

**Thank the mother..**

## 5- PEDIATRICS — COMMUNICATION SKILLS..

*Trick: 'You have to use the country **native** language..'*

### Diabetes mellitus ' How to Use a Glucometer ':

Greet the mother & the patient,
Introduce yourself,
Take permission..

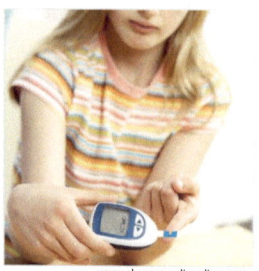
www.abcnewsradioonline.com

Obtain a glucometer and test strips..

Wash the child hands thoroughly, including the area from which you are going to draw blood..

Place alcohol on a cotton ball..

Place a test strip into the slot provided on the glucometer..

Swab the area you are going to use to draw your sample from with the cotton ball..
 *(Alcohol evaporates rapidly so there's no need to dry the area. That will just re-contaminate it )..*

Wait for the readout on the diabetic glucometer to tell you to put the drop of blood on the strip..

Use the lancet provided with the diabetic glucose meter and prick the area for the sample..

Place a drop of blood on the test strip <u>without the finger touching the strip</u> & if touched the reading may be wrong *(and this is one of the techniqual errors that may occur)..*

Wait for results..

Read and record your results..
 **You have to plot a chart** *(date & time, blood sugar reading & insulin dose)..*

**Thank the mother..**

*Trick: You can ask the mother if she has any questions, that will help you to remember if you forget any important information in the communication skills OSCE station or in your daily practical life..*

## 5- PEDIATRICS    COMMUNICATION SKILLS..

Trick: 'You have to use the country **native** language.'

### Lumbar puncture:

Greet the mother & the patient,
Introduce yourself,
Take permission..

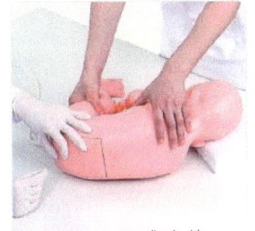

We suspect that your child has meningitis, which is a curable disease & its treatment is available..

But, to diagnose the disease we need a cerebral spinal fluid by a lumbar puncture.. it is simple, not danger prick like any prick of injection in the other body parts..

**If she refuse..**

The disease is dangerous and has a lot of complications like seizure, increase the intracranial pressure, paralysis & with time may loss his vision, hearing or even become mental retarded *(choose the simple complications & easy to understand by the mother)*..

**If she refuses.. ' my relative was agree to do a lumbar puncture to his son which is know paralyzed !!, the mother said '..**

O.K., believe me this is completely wrong, these are only rumors.. it is from other reason & not from the lumbar puncture itself..

**If she insist to refuse the lumbar puncture..**

O.K., we will give him an empirical treatment for 2 weeks, but we don't know whether it is the appropriate one or not (we will choose the most appropriate one).. and we follow his condition..  ***BUT, believe me → the lumbar puncture is a right choice for his condition at this time (it is simple but worthy test)..***

**Thank the mother..**

# 5- PEDIATRICS    COMMUNICATION SKILLS..

Trick: *You have to use the country native language.*

### How to Sterilize & Prepare Baby Bottles:

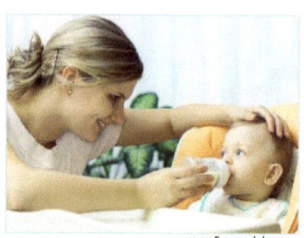

Greet the mother,
Introduce yourself,
Take permission..

Wash the bottle & nipple using water, table salt & with 2 brushes large one for bottle & small one for nipple..

Place a pot, filled with water, on the stove and turn the heat on to high till boiling..

Place the bottle in the water for **10 min.** (15 min. if glass bottle), then add the nipple to the water for **5 min.** → So, the full time is *15 min.* (20 min. if glass bottle)..

Turn off the stove, and wait till the water become cold.. (don't use cold water)..

Close the bottle and put it in the refrigerator..

**When you want to prepare a milk baby bottle:**
First, put the **water** in the bottle *then* add the milk..
*Never* dilute the milk..**!!**

*Once no. calculation:*
The ideal method (*according to weight*)..
Each 1 kg. need 100 k. calorie → So, **weight** X 100 = *no. of k. cal. / day*
There are 20 k.cal. in each ounce → So, **no. of k.cal.** / 20 = no. of ounce / day

For example.. the child weight is **4 kg..**
So, 4 X 100 = 400 k. cal. / day → 400 / 20 = **20 ounce / day**

The practical method (*according to weight*)..
**Weight** X 5 = No. of ounce
So, the previous example → 4 X 5 = **20 ounce / day**

[ Ideally, the no. of bottles = no. feedings / day ]..
And definitely, it is depend on the economic status of the family..

You may need to mention the advantages & disadvantages of the breast and bottle feedings to the baby and the mother..
(*please, see the next page*..)

Trick: Each one OUNCE = 30 mL

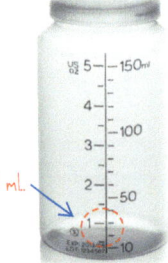

*Therapeutic formula:*
Soya based, CHO free milk & hydrolyzed protein formula
For specific medical purposes (*like 1° & 2° lactase deficiency, galactosemia, fructosemia & cow milk protein intolerance*)..

**Thank the mother..**

## 5- PEDIATRICS — COMMUNICATION SKILLS..

Trick: *'You have to use the country native language..'*

### Breast feeding:

Greet the mother,

Introduce yourself,

Take permission..

The breast feeding is better than bottle feeding because the advantages *to the baby as well as to the mother..*

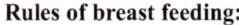

And don't forget, it is *easier, safer, cheaper & readily available..*

No milk allergy, has antimicrobial property, keep its gut sterile, and is consider the first natural vaccine you can give to the baby..

Also has proteins, fat, carbohydrates, water, vitamins & minerals..

Emotionally satisfactory for the mother & it gives feeling of security to the baby..

### Rules of breast feeding:

Demand feeding & baby freedom..

↑↑ no. of feeding at night..

He should finish one breast then go to the other..

Rooming in or bedding in the same room..

*There are **no** real disadvantages of breast milk*, only we need to acknowledge them and deal with them immediately *(e.g.: inadequate lactation, demand maternal proximity, social life acceptance & treating cracked nipples by teaching the mother the technique of feeding)..*

### Contraindication of breast feeding: ' *most of them temporary* '

In mother: Sever systemic disease (acute heart failure, hepatitis B, neoplasia..etc)

Acute infection (active T.B., malaria, local bilateral breast abscesses..etc)

Insanity & uncontrolled epilepsy..

Sever inverted nipple not responding to local treatment..

In the baby: Iinborn error of metabolism (*absolute C.I.*)..

Sever physical abnormalities as bilateral cleft palate & cleft lip..

Weak & premature infant..    Sever dyspnoea as RDS & H.F.

Cerebral anoxia..

**Thank the mother..**

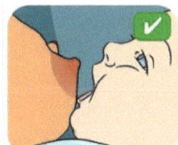 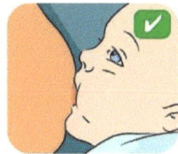 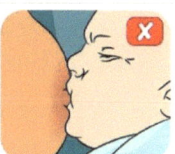

To start the feed, hold baby so her chest is touching your chest, her nose should be in line with your nipple. Gently brush your nipple from her nose to her upper lip – this will encourage her to open her mouth wide.

When her mouth is wide open, **bring baby to your breast** keeping your hands across her back and shoulders. When she attaches, most of the areola will be in her mouth and her chin will be tucked into the breast. When she's feeding well, she'll suck deeply and regularly, and you'll hear her swallowing.

When baby is not correctly attached and just sucks the nipple, feeding is painful, nipples can become damaged and the breast won't be properly drained. If baby hasn't attached correctly, stop, take her off the breast as shown below and try again.

www.abc.net.au

## 5- PEDIATRICS — COMMUNICATION SKILLS..

Trick: *'You have to use the country native language..'*

### Oral rehydration solution (O.R.S.):

Greet the mother,

Introduce yourself,

Take permission..

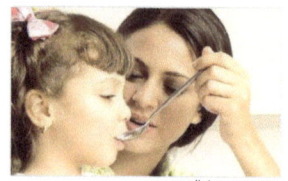

www.media1.onsugar.com

Your son has diarrhea.. but without dehydration yet..

So, *no* need for admission.. but you have to give him this solution *(Dextrolyte solution)*..

The child must continue his feeding (if he is breast fed to continue on feeding him with small frequent sips, if he is bottle fed to give fewer ounces but frequent times & if he is on diet to give him soft easily digestible diet in small amount and frequent times)..

Dissolve one pack in 1 liter of boiled water & wait till the water become cold then add the *Dextrolyte* solution..

It is given by spoon gradually to avoid acute gastric distension which causes vomiting & it is used for 24 h only..

For *below 24 months* → we give **50-100cc** of O.R.S. for each bowel motion passed and if the age *2-10 years* → we give **100-200 cc**..

If he vomits, we *wait for 10 minutes* and **then continue** giving the O.R.S by spoon but more slowly..

You have to bring the child to the 1° health care center if he is still having diarrhea after 2 days

**Thank the mother..**

---

### Uses of O.R.S (DEXTROLYTE):
- It is given in acute diarrhea with **no dehydration** state to prevent dehydration..
- Also given for rehydration in **some dehydration** (mild to moderate) state..
- It is given for the **ongoing loss**..

### Composition of O.R.S:
- NaCl → 3.5 g/l, NaHCO$_3$ → 2.5 g/l, KCl → 1.5 g/l, Glucose 20 g/l..

### Concentration of O.R.S:
- Na$^+$ → 90 mmol/l, HCO$_3^-$ → 30 mmol/l, K$^+$ → 20 mmol/l, Cl$^-$ → 80 mmol/l & Glucose → 111 mmol/l..

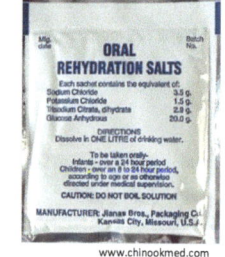

www.chinookmed.com

## 5- PEDIATRICS     COMMUNICATION SKILLS..

Trick: *'You have to use the country native language..'*

### Enuresis:

Greet the mother,

Introduce yourself,

Take permission..

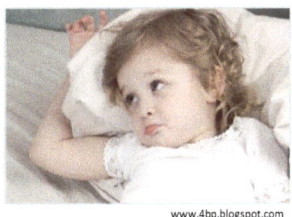

Doing nothing or punishing the child are both common responses to bedwetting. Neither helps.

You should reassure your child that bedwetting is common and can be helped.

Start by making sure that your child goes to the bathroom at normal times during the day and evening and does not hold urine for long periods of time.

Be sure that the child goes to the bathroom before going to sleep. You can reduce the amount of fluid the child drinks a few hours before bedtime, but this alone is not a treatment for bedwetting. You should not restrict fluids excessively.

Reward your child for dry nights. Some families use a chart or diary that the child can mark each morning.

Bedwetting alarms are another method that can be used along with reward systems. The alarms are small and readily available without a prescription at many stores.
The alarm wakes the child or parent when the child starts to urinate, so the child can get up and use the bathroom.

*A prescription medication called DDAVP (desmopressin) is available to treat bedwetting.*

*Tricyclic antidepressants (most often imipramine) can also help with bedwetting.*

**Thank the mother..**

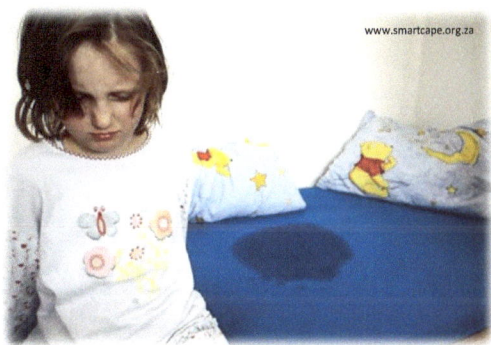

**Don't forget -** You should *reassure* the parents & the child that bedwetting is common and can be helped..

# 5- PEDIATRICS — COMMUNICATION SKILLS..

*Trick: 'You have to use the country **native** language..'*

## Vaccination:

Greet the mother & introduce yourself,
Take permission..

Ask about → *Age* &
   *The previous vaccination..*

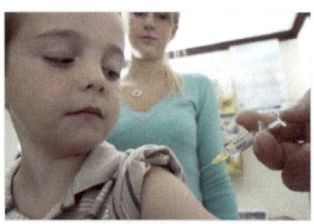

*Vaccination schedule in Iraq:*

At birth → BCG,   OPV-0,   HBV-1
2 mo. completed → DTP-1,   OPV-1,   HBV-2   *+ Rota virus & H. influenza vaccine*
4 mo. completed → DTP-2,   OPV-2,            *+ Rota virus & H. influenza vaccine*
6 mo. completed → DTP-3,   OPV-3,   HBV-3   *+ Rota virus & H. influenza vaccine*
*9 mo.* completed → **Measles..**
*15 mo.* completed → **MMR..**
18 mo. completed → DTP , OPV (**booster no.1**) + Vitamin A 200 I.U.
4-6 years → DTP , OPV (**booster no.2**) + MMR 2

What if a child misses a shot ?

In the First visit → DTP-1, OPV-1, HBV-1   *+ Rota virus & H. influenza vaccine*
   (± BCG)..

1 mo. later → MMR..
1-2 mo. later → DTP-2, OPV-2, HBV-2   *+ Rota virus & H. influenza vaccine*
1-2 mo. later → DTP-3, OPV-3, HBV-3   *+ Rota virus & H. influenza vaccine*
**15-18 mo.** later → DTP , OPV (**booster**)..

*NOTE: BCG vaccine is given to the baby in the first year to protect him from miliary T.B. & T.B. encephalitis → So, after the 1st year is of **NO benefit**..*

Vaccination checklist: *(Be sure to ask these questions before giving the vaccines)..*

- Is your child **sick today** ? (*more than a common cold, earache ..etc*)..
- Does your child have any **sever** (life-threatening) **allergies** ?
- Has your child ever had **severe reaction after a vaccination** ?
- Does your child have a **weakened immune system** (bec. of disease or medication) ?
- Has your child **gotten a transfusion** or any other blood product, recently ?
  *(if yes → wait 3 months..)..*
- Has your child ever had **convulsion** or **any kind of nervous system problem** ?
- Does your child not seem to be **developing normally** ?

## 5- PEDIATRICS  COMMUNICATION SKILLS..

*General contraindication for vaccination:*
- Serious allergic reaction (*e.g.: anaphylaxis after a previous vaccine dose*)..
- Serious allergic reaction (*e.g.: anaphylaxis*) to a vaccine component..
- Moderate to severe illness with or without fever..

*FALSE contraindication for vaccination:*
- Mild acute illness with low grade fever or mild diarrhea..
- Mild to moderate local reaction (*soreness, redness or swelling*) after a dose of an injectable antigen..
- Current antimicrobial therapy..
- Prematurity..
- Malnutrition..
- Breast feeding..
- Pregnancy of mother or household contact..
- History of penicillin or other non specific allergy..
- Family $H_x$ of convulsion in child considered for pertussis or measles vaccination..
- Current antimicrobial therapy..

Vaccination in immunecompromised child: (*e.g.: with cancer or taking steroid*)..
- B̶C̶G̶, M̶M̶R̶, O̶P̶V̶ & R̶o̶t̶a̶ v. (*live attenuated*) → are CONTRAINDICATED..
- Give **HBV**..

Vaccination in pregnancy:
- B̶C̶G̶, M̶M̶R̶, O̶P̶V̶ & R̶o̶t̶a̶ v. (*live attenuated*) → are CONTRAINDICATED..
- Give **tetanus toxoid**..
  (At the 4$^{th}$ & the 5$^{th}$ months of pregnancy,
  then after 6 mo., 1 year, & 2 years)..

Why we give the vaccine according to the schedule ?

Answer: because at this time the immune system is mature enough to make the antibodies.. otherwise it is with no benefit..

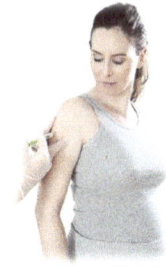

AT THE END: thank the mother..

# 5- PEDIATRICS — COMMUNICATION SKILLS..

Trick: *'You have to use the country native language..'*

**Vaccines:** *(To be oriented..!!)*

### BCG:

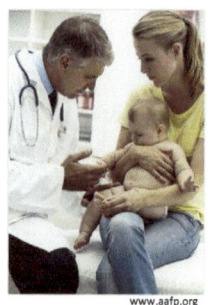

Is given as a single injection..
(intradermal + left side + at deltoid m. insertion).

A local abscess may form (BCG-oma) that may ulcerate & often requires treatment with antibiotic (erythromycin)..

Adverse effects → Keloids, large ugly scar (*main adverse effect*),
Suppurative lymphadenitis (less common)..

If the mother refuse to give it to his child → *Explain to her that his child may become at risk of Miliary T.B. or T.B. encephalitis which are dangerous complication & lead to death..*

### OPV:

Is given as oral drpos..

Adverse effects → on very rare occasions has been associated with paralysis (1 case per 750,000 vaccine recipient).. '**Don't** *mention this to the mother*'

If the mother refuse to give it to his child → *Explain to her that his child may become at risk of paralysis (may become unable to walk) & may affect on his respiration (may lead to death)..*

### Hepatitis B vaccine:

Is given intramuscular as a three-dose series..
If the mother refuse to give it to his child → *Explain to her that his child may become at risk of hepatitis virus (which affect the liver functions)..*

### DTP:

Is given intramuscular (0.5 ml)..
Adverse effects → minor: redness, swelling & painless nodule at the site of injection..
moderate: ongoing crying, high fever (up to 40) & unusual screaming..
severe: serious allergic reaction, seizures & encephalitis (very rare)..

If the mother refuse to give it to his child → *Explain to her that his child may become at risk of* : Pertussis: cough & respiratory problems → pneumonia (*most dangerous complication*)..
Diphtheria: may lead to respiratory & heart failure..
Tetanus: fever then spasms → may affect the respiratory system..

## 5- PEDIATRICS — COMMUNICATION SKILLS..

*Trick: 'You have to use the country native language.'*

### MMR:

Greet the mother & introduce yourself,
Take permission..

Is given subcutaneously in two doses..

Adverse effects → fever & rash in 10% of children, 10 days after vaccine administration..
Transient arthritis & thrombocytopenia..

What are the benefits from this vaccine ?
  To protect the baby from measles, mumps & rubella..
  *Rubella is given to ♀, not to protect her from rubella only but to prevent congenital rubella in pregnancy (to the baby if she get pregnant)..*

If the mother refuse to give it to his child → *Explain to her that his child may become at risk of:*

  Rubella: Cause the same adverse effects of the vaccine but the commonest are arthralgia & arthritis..
  Measles: Cause fever, rash, influenza like symptoms, cough ..etc
      The commonest complication is otitis media but the dangerous one is 1° or 2° pneumonia..
  Mumps: Cause fever, influenza like symptoms, parotitis..etc
      The dangerous complication is meningitis.
      Orchitis is common in ♂ patients..

**Thank the mother..**

---

### in / ARABIC /:

BCG = / LiL TADARON /,
OPV = / Li SHALAL al ATFAAL /,
H.B. vaccine = / Li ELTEHAB AL KABAD AL VAiROSee /

DTP → D (Diphtheria) = / AL KhANAK /,
    T (Tetanus) = / AL KOZAZZ /,
    P (Pertussis) = / AL So'AAL AL DEEKi /

MMR → M (Measles) = / AL HASBah /,
    M (Mumps) = / AL NOKAF /,
    R (Rubella) = / AL HASBah AL ALMANiAh /

Rota virus = / AL virus AL DAWAAR /,
*H. influenza vaccine* = / LiL MUSTADMIA AL NAZLiAA /,

## 5- PEDIATRICS — INVESTIGATIONS..

**Normal values:**

WBC = 4 – 11    X $10^9$/L,

Hb = 11 – 16    X g/dL,

Platelets = 150 – 400    X $10^9$/L,

PCV = 37% – 47% in ♀   [ Hb = (PCV-1) / 33 ]

Reticulocytes → < 2%

PT = 12 – 14    sec.
PTT = 30 – 45    sec.
TT = 10 – 13    sec.    *' TT = Thrombin Time '*
BT = 4 – 8    min.

Reticulocytes = <2%

## MCV:
*80 - 95*

**Less:** *(microcytic hypochromic)*
- Iron deficiency anemia
- Thalassemia (major → Hb F >50%)
- Lead poisoning

**Normal:** *(normocytic normochromic)*
- Hemolytic anemia
- Blood loss
- Renal disease
- ..etc

**More:** *(macrocytic..)*
- Megaloblastic anemia
- B12 & folate deficiency

## Cerebrospinal fluid (CSF) analysis:

### Normal values:

Cells → <5      cell/mm$^2$   (75% lymphocytes),

Proteins =   20 – 45   mg/dL,

Glucose →  > 50%   mg/dL    (75% of serum glucose)

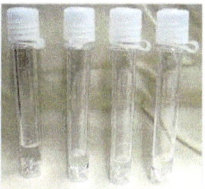

### Meningitis:

|  | Pressure | Cells | Proteins | Glucose |
|---|---|---|---|---|
| *Acute bacterial m.* | N. or ↑↑ | ↑↑ polymorph. | ↑↑ | ↓↓↓ |
| *Viral m.* | N. | ↑ Lymphocytes | N. / ↑↑ | N. |
| *T.B.* | N. or ↑↑ | ↑ Lymphocytes | ↑↑ | ↓↓ |
| *Partial R$_x$ bacterial m.* | N. | ↑ Mononuclear | ↑↑ | N. |

*N. = normal, m. = meningitis*

### Guillain barré syndrome:

Albuminocytological dissociation (if the protein is only ↑↑ + oligoclonal band)..

## 5- PEDIATRICS — INVESTIGATIONS..

### Nephrotic syndrome Vs. Glumerilunephritis:

| **Nephrotic syndrome..** | **Glumerilunephritis..** |
|---|---|
| 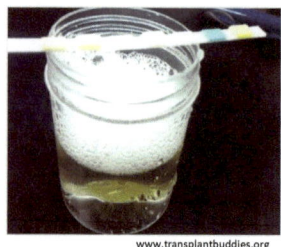 | 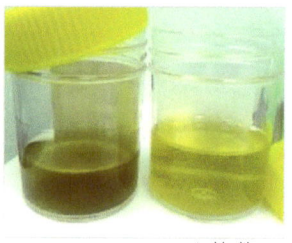 |
| Normal color, frothy.. | Red, macroscopic hematuria.. |
| Proteins: +++ / ++++ (heavy proteinuria) | + |
| Casts: X | present |
| RBCs: X | > 5 (hematuria) |

**NOTE:**

Normal serum albumin = 60 – 80 g/L..

## 5- PEDIATRICS — INVESTIGATIONS..

Trick:

This is the easiest way to memorize the HEMATOLOGY investigations, in general, not only in pediatrics.. !!

|  | **ITP** | **TTP** | **E.T.** |
|---|---|---|---|
| *Platelets* | ↓ (< 80 × $10^9$) | ↓ (< 20 × $10^9$) | ↑ (600-2500 × $10^9$) |
| *B.T.* | ↑ | ↑ | N. |
| *PT* | N. | N. | N. |
| *PTT* | N. | N. | N. |
| *Bone marrow* | N. or ↑↑ megakaryocyte | N. or ↑↑ cellularity | megakaryocytosis |
| Other $I_x$ | Antiplatelet Ab +ve.. | WBC ↑↑ gingival biopsy | WBC ↑↑ Abnormal platelets Hb urea |

* N. = normal, E.T. = Essential thrombocytopenia..

|  | **Haemphilia A** | **VWD** |
|---|---|---|
| *Platelets* | N. | N. |
| *B.T.* | N. | ↑ |
| *PT* | N. | N. |
| *PTT* | ↑ | ↑ |
| Other $I_x$ | ↓ Factor VIII ↓ VWF | ↓ Factor VIII ↓↓ VWF |

**Vitamin K deficiency:** PT → ↑↑ , PTT → ↑ , platelets → N. , B.T → N.

Liver diseases & DIC: ALL $I_x$ → ABNORMAL

Trick: Pancytopenia = ↓↓ platelets, ↓↓ WBC, ↓↓ Hb. → For example, in aplastic anemia, leukemia & Kala-azar..

# 5- PEDIATRICS — FOLLOW UP CHARTS..

## Follow up charts:

### Patient with meningitis:

General examination (especially the consciousness & posture)..
Vital signs..
Fontanelle, OFC, pupil & fundoscopy..
Cranial nn. examination (especially the $6^{th}$)..
Meningeal signs..
Upper & lower limbs neurological examination..
Input & output fluid & weight..
Any new investigation should be checked..

### Patient with nephrotic syndrome:

Edema..
Urine output..
Weight..
Vital signs..
General wellbeing..
Steroid S.E..
Any complication (infection, thrombosis & hyperlipidemia)..
G.U.E & serum albumin..

### Patient with Guillain Barré syndrome:

General examination..
Vital signs..
Upper & lower limbs neurological examination..
Cranial nn. Examination (especially the $6^{th}$)..
History of chocking or regurgitation..
Assessment for bulbar involvement..
Reflexes & autonomic dysfunction (such as profuse sweating, palpitation & postural hypotension)
Sphincter disturbances..

### Diabetes mellitus:

Name, age, date & time
Body weight & surface area..
Pulse rate & B.P..
PH, RBS, S. electrolytes, insulin dose..
Fluid input, output & signs of cerebral edema..
Any other notes..

# 5- PEDIATRICS
## DEVELOPMENT MADE VERY EASY ' by Dr. M.O.M '..

Developmental milestones:

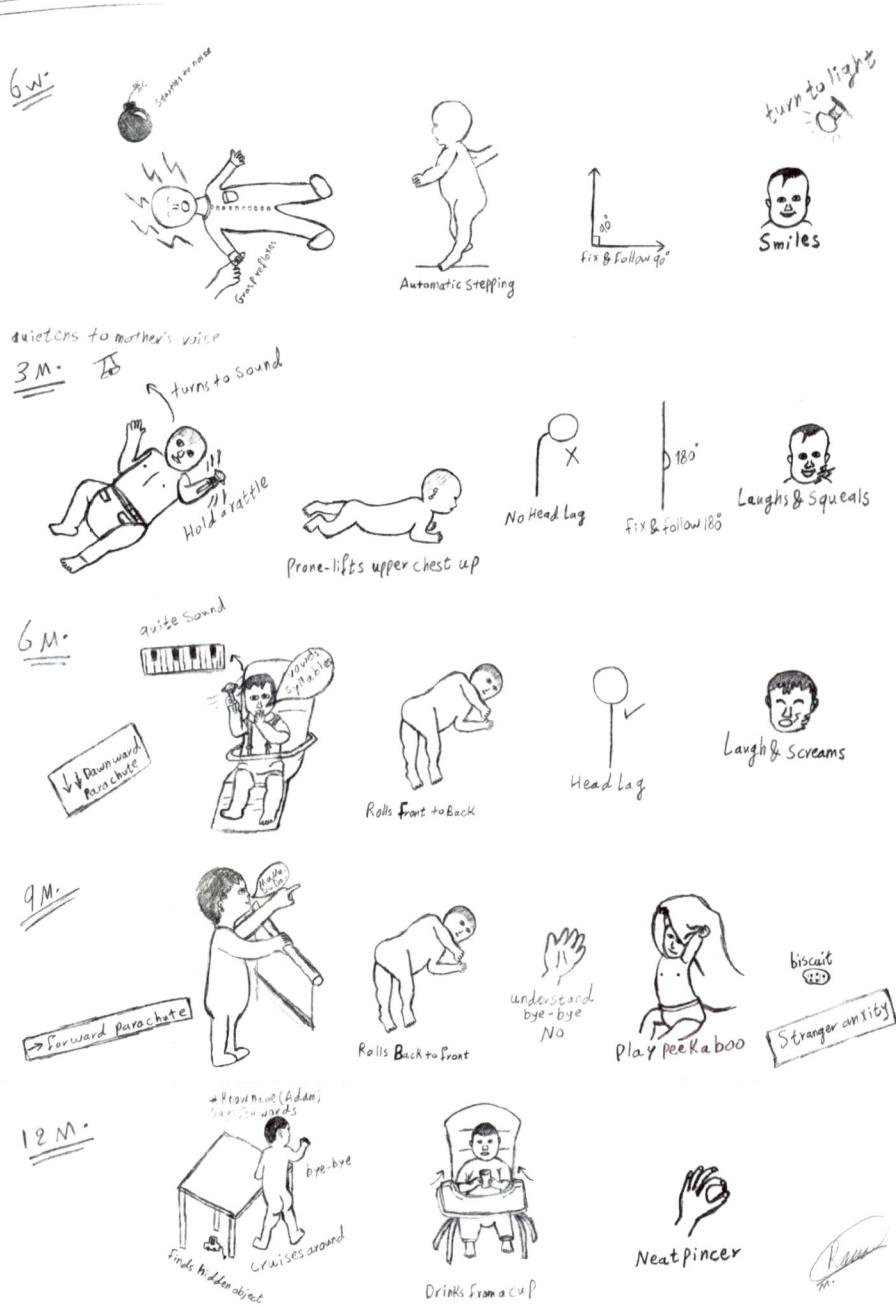

## 5- PEDIATRICS — DEVELOPMENT MADE VERY EASY ' by Dr. M.O.M '..

**15 M:**

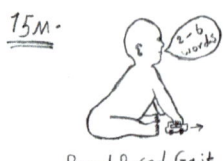
Broad Based Gait

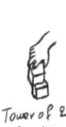
Tower of 2 Bricks

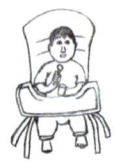
Uses cup & spoon

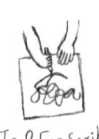
To & Fro Scribble

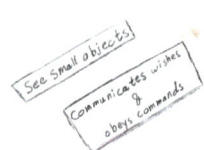
- 2-6 words
- See small objects
- Communicates wishes & obeys commands

**18 M:**

- 6-14 words
- Hand preference

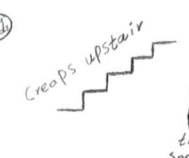
Creeps upstairs

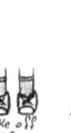
Takes off socks & shoes

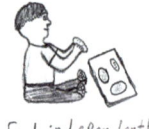
Feed independently

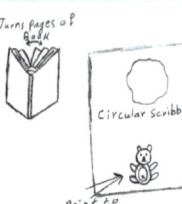
Turns pages of book

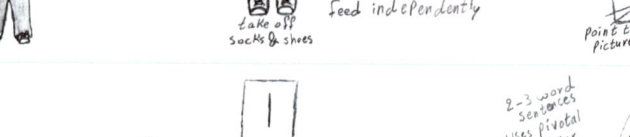
Circular Scribble — Point to picture

**2 y:**

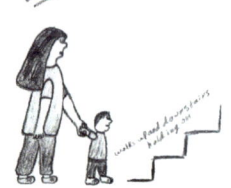
Walks up & down stairs holding on

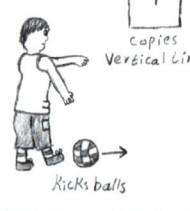
Kicks balls

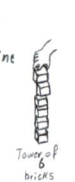
Copies Vertical Line

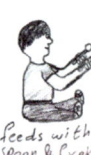
Tower of 6 bricks

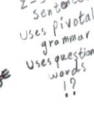
Feeds with spoon & fork

- 2-3 word sentences
- Uses pivotal grammar
- Uses question words (What?)

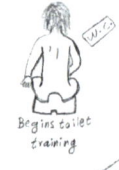
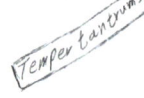
Begins toilet training — Temper tantrums

**3 y:**

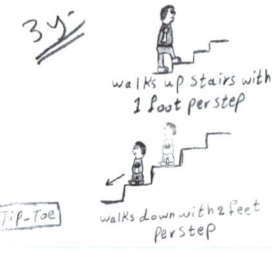
Walks up stairs with 1 foot per step
Walks down with 2 feet per step
Tip-Toe

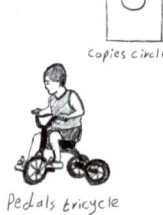
Pedals tricycle

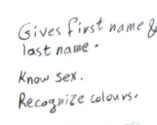
Copies circle

- Gives first name & last name.
- Knows sex.
- Recognize colours.

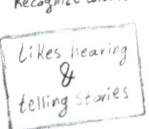
Likes hearing & telling stories

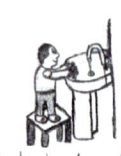
Washes hands and brushes teeth — Eats with fork & spoon

**4 y:**

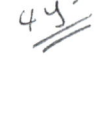
Hops

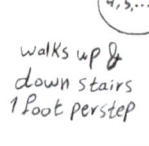
Walks up & down stairs 1 foot per step — 1, 2, 3, 4, 5, ...10

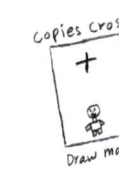
Copies cross — Draw man

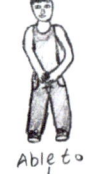
Able to undress

**5 y:**

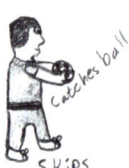
Skips — Catches ball

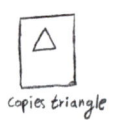
Copies triangle

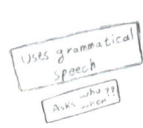
Uses grammatical speech — Asks who? when?

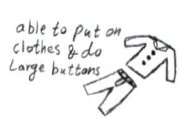
Able to put on clothes & do large buttons

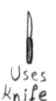

Uses knife

## 5- PEDIATRICS — DRUGS ' ESSENTIALS NOTES '..

### DRUGS ' ESSENTIALS NOTES ' :

#### Diazepam amp. ( Valium ) :

**Indication :** In stop convulsions
*( Not to treat it .. So, it is used in E.R. not at home )*

**Main S/E :** Respiratory depression
*( So, monitor the respiratory rate )*

**Dose :** 0.1 – 0.3 mg/kg/dose , Given by slow diluted I.V.
*( If there is no I.V. access , you can give it rectally )*
*Can be repeated 3 times in status epilepticus*

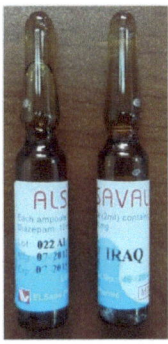

#### Phenytoin ( Epanutin ) amp. & Phenobarbital ( Luminal ) amp. :

**Indication :** In status epilepticus (2nd line of Rx )
In convulsion *( Whatever the cause )*
Head trauma
Subarachnoid hemorrhage

**Main S/E :** Change in the level of consciousness
Nausea & vomiting

**Dose :** Loading dose 15 – 20 mg/kg/dose   I.V. slow infusion
Maintenance dose 5 mg/kg in 2 divided doses   I.V. slow infusion

*Compatible with N/S , never give it with G/W*

**Note :** Whenever patient more than 6 years comes with fever , photophobia & convulsion .. this is unlikely to be febrile convulsion because age of febrile convulsion is *( 5 months – 6 months )*

**Note :** Phenytoin → When we need to remain the patient conscious ( ex. Meningitis )
Phenobarbital → When sedation is needed ( Cerebral palsy & hypoglycemic fit )

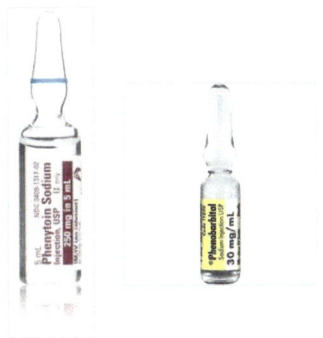

## Hydrocortisone vial & Dexamethasone amp ( Decadron amp.):

**Action:** H.C. is more rapid ( So, used in acute stage like *Asthma & Anaphylaxis* )
Dexamethasone is more potent & longer duration

**Main S/E :** Hypertension
Hyperglycemia
Gastric upset
Paresthesia ( For Decadron )

**Dose :** H.C. → 10 mg/kg/day I.V. ( Can be repeated )
either Once ( 10 mg/kg ),
Twice ( 5 then 5 mg/kg ) or
Thrice ( 3 , 3 then 3 mg/kg )

Dexamethasone → 0.1 – 0.3 mg/kg in 4 divided doses I.V.
0.6 mg/kg/dose I.V.
*( Used in meningitis to decrease cerebral edema )*

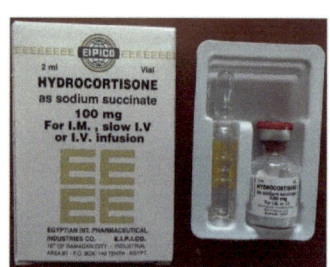
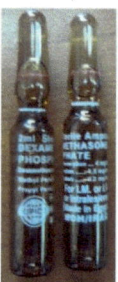

## Sodium Bicarbonate NaHCO$_3$ 8.4% ( and there is 7% & 9.5% ) amp. :

**Indication :** In severe acidosis such as DKA &
Renal failure *( When PH is less than 7.2 )*

**Main S/E :** Hypokalemia
Hypoglycemia
Cerebral edema

**Dose :** 1cc/kg/dose 4 times daily I.V. slow
*( But not more than 25 mg/dose )*

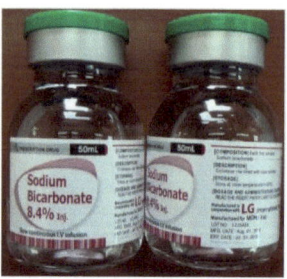

## 5- PEDIATRICS — DRUGS ' ESSENTIALS NOTES '..

### Metoclopramide ( Plasil ) amp. :

**Note :** It is dopamine antagonist

**Indication :** For nausea & vomiting

**Main S/E :** Oculogyric crises
  *( So, it is used with caution in pediatric & treated with Allermin & Atropine )*

**Dose :** 0.1-0.2 mg/kg/dose I.V. or I.M.

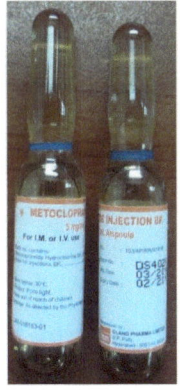

### Epinephrine ( Adrenaline ) amp. :

**Note :** It is sympathomimetic drug

**Indication :** Anaphylaxis ( given S.C. )
  Cardiac standstill ( I.V. or Intracardiac)
  Anaphylactic shock as ( S.C. )
  Sever laryngeal edema in case of croup

**Main S/E :** Tachycardia
  Hypertension

**Dose :** 0.01 mg/kg/dose

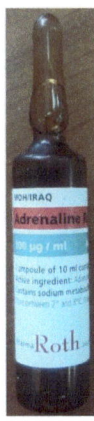

### Aminophylline amp. :

**Indication :** : In severe asthma not responding to salbutamol & H.C. as bronchodilator

**Main S/E :** Tachycardia
  Dysrhythmia
  Nausea & Vomiting

**Dose :** 3-5 mg/kg continuous I.V. slow infusion in **30 cc G/W 5%** over 1/2 h
  *or* 3 times bolus 5 mg/kg/hr

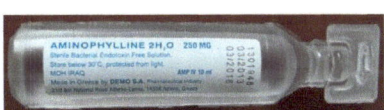

# 5- PEDIATRICS — DRUGS ' ESSENTIALS NOTES '..

### Furosemide ( Lasix ) amp. :

**Note :** It is loop diuretics

**Indication :** In fluid overload including
  *Over-replacement in treatment of dehydration*
  *Edema*
  *Hypertension*

**Main S/E :** Hypovolemia
  Hypocalcaemia
  Hypokalemia
  *Hyperuricemia*

**Dose :** 1-2 mg/kg/dose I.V. ( Can be repeated 3 times )

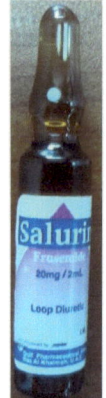

### Tranexamic acid ( Cyklokapron ) amp. :

**Note :** Antifibrinolytic agent

**Indication :** In mucosal bleeding ( gum , nasal , GIT , vaginal , uterine .. etc. )

**Main S/E :** Thrombosis
  Hypotension
  Nausea & Vomiting

**C.I. :** In case of hematuria
  ( Because it may cause obstructive
  uropathy & acute renal failure )

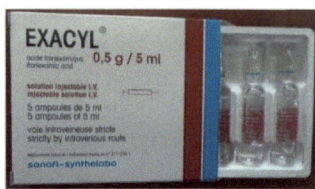

**Dose :** 45 mg/kg /day in 3 divided doses slow I.V. infusion with N/S

### Hyosine-N-Butylbromide ( Buscopan ) amp. :

**Note :** Anticholinergic drug

**Indication :** In acute spasm of bowel
  ( Colicky abdominal pain )

**Main S/E :** Lazy bowel syndrome
  Paralytic ileus

**Dose :** 0.1 – 0.2 mg/kg/dose I.V.

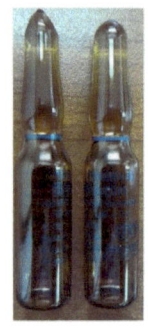

## 5- PEDIATRICS     DRUGS ' ESSENTIALS NOTES '..

### Vit. K ' Phytomenadione ' amp. :

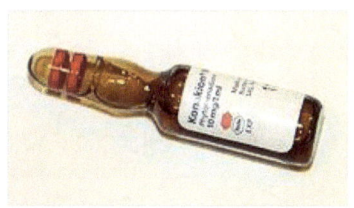

**Indication :** To decrease the risk of bleeding in neonate after birth *(hemorrhagic disease of new born at day 2-7 of life )*

       Bleeding due to chronic liver disease

**Dose :** Therapeutic → 5 mg/day single dose daily until the bleeding stops
       Prophylactic → 1 mg/day
       I.M. or I.V

       In liver disease is given in alternate days with plasma

### Salbutamol ( Ventolin solution ) :

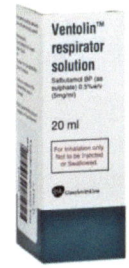
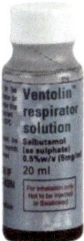

**Indication :** In acute bronchospasm
           *( it is act on smooth muscle of bronchus causing relaxation )*

**Main S/E :** Tachycardia
           Tremor

**Dose :** 0.6 mg/kg in 24 hr
       Ventolin nebulizer → *Add 0.5 cc Salbutamol solution in 1.5 cc N/S & put it in nebulizer ( can repeat it 3 times )*

### Ranitidin amp. (Zantac) & Cimetidine amp. (Tagamet):

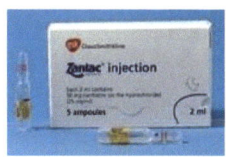

**Note :** It is $H_2$ blocker

**Indication :** Gastric ulcer
          GERD
          Stress ulcer
          Esophageal varices

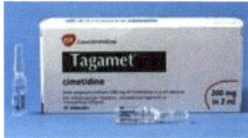

**Dose :** Ranitidin 1-2 mg/kg/dose I.V. × 2
       Cimetidine 10 mg/kg/dose I.V. × 2

## 5- PEDIATRICS — DRUGS ' ESSENTIALS NOTES '..

### Sodium stibogluconate ( Pentostam) :

**Indication :** Anti-leishmaniasis

**Main S/E :** Nausea & vomiting
           Abdominal pain
           Elevated liver enzymes
           Fever
           ECG changes

**Dose :** 20 mg/kg/day once daily for 20 days
       I.M. or *I.V. infusion with filter*

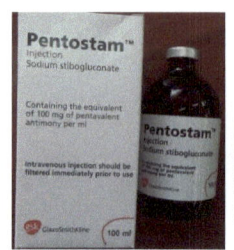
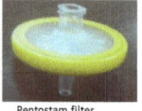
Pentostam filter

### Potassium (Kcl) amp. :

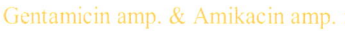

**Indication :** For treatment of Hypokalemia
             DKA
             Dehydration with repeated vomiting
             Paralytic ileus

**Dose :** 1 ml/kg
        Each ml ( cc ) = 2 meq Kcl
        So, each kg needs 1 cc .. For example, we have 10 kg infant who needs 1000 cc fluid , we add 10 ccs Kcl to 1000 cc fluid ( 2 pints ) but never put more than 10 cc of Kcl in one liter .. *( So, do not exceeds 5 cc / pint of fluid )*

### Gentamicin amp. & Amikacin amp. :

**Note :** It is antibiotic (Aminoglycoside group ) ..
       Strong against G-ve and may use for G+ve

**Indication :** UTI
             Gastroenteritis

**Dose :** Gentamicin amp 3-5 mg/kg/day 2 divided doses
       Amikacin amp 15 mg/kg/day in 2 divided doses
       I.M. or I.V.

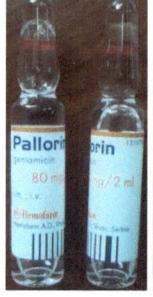
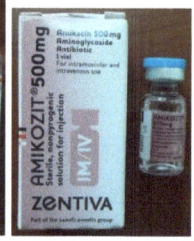

## 5- PEDIATRICS — DRUGS ' ESSENTIALS NOTES '..

### Cefotaxime ( Claforan ) , Ceftriaxone ( Rocephin ) , Ceftazidime ( Fortum ) Vial :

**Note :** There are Cephalosporins group of ABTs

All have the same efficacy on Gram +ve microorganisms *but there efficacy on Gram –ve increase respectively ( Fortum > Rocephin > Claforan )*

Ceftazidim is a potent anti-pseudomonal ABT

**Dose :**

*Claforan* 100 mg/kg/day in 2 divided doses

*Ceftriaxone* 50-100 mg/kg/day in 2 divided doses

**Dose :** *I.M. or I.V. infusion*

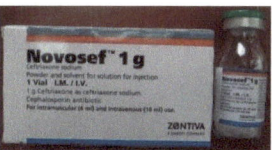

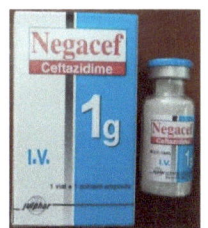 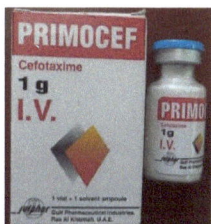

### Calcium Gluconate 10% amp. :

**Indication :** Hypocalcaemia

Hyperkalemia *( To protect the heart )*

Renal failure

**Dose :** 1 cc/kg/day by I.V. infusion in **G/W** per 6 hrs

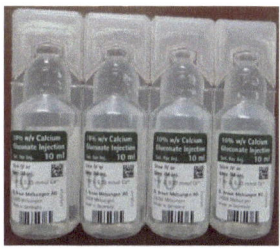

### Chlorpheniramine ( Allermine ) amp. :

**Note :** Antihistamine

**Dose :** 1 mg/kg/dose I.M. or I.V.

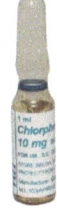

## 5- PEDIATRICS — DRUGS ' ESSENTIALS NOTES '..

### Atropine amp. :

**Indication :** For Bradycardia caused by Organophosphorus poisoning

**Dose :** 0.01 mg/kg I.V.

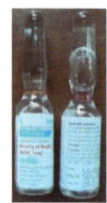

### Ampiclox vial :

**Note :** It is Ampicillin and Cloxacillin

**C.I. :** in Penicillin allergy

**Dose :** 200 mg/kg/day in 4 divided doses I.M or I.V.

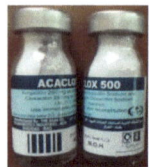

### Metronidazole ( Flagyl ) bottle :

**Indication :** For Anaerobes & Parasites

**Dose :** 5-7 mg/kg/dose X 3
      ( 1.5 cc/kg/dose X 3 ) I.V.

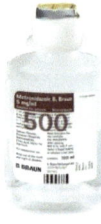

### Acetaminophen ( **Antipyrol** ) syrup :

**Indication :** For pain & fever relief

**Dose :** 10-15 mg/kg/dose X 3  oral

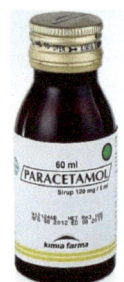

### Digioxen amp. :

**Digitalization :** 0.02 – 0.04 mg/kg/dose
                1/2 dose → (1$^{st}$) 8 hr.
                1/4 dose → (2$^{nd}$) 8 hr.
                1/4 dose → (3$^{rd}$) 8 hr.

**Maintenance :** 0.005 – 0.01 mg/kg/day
              ( LAST DOSE / 2 )

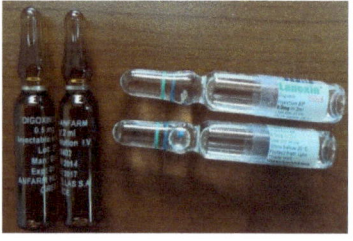

## 5- PEDIATRICS — DRUGS ' ESSENTIALS NOTES '..

### INSULIN vial :

Soluble :

YELLOW VIAL, clear solution

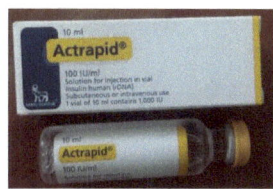

Lente:

LIGHT BLUE or GREEN vial, cloudy

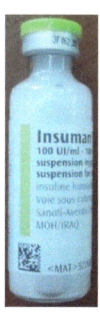

Mixed:

Brown vial, cloudy , written on it  *30 \ 70 ( 30% soluble + 70% Lente )*

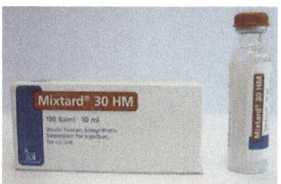

### GLUCAGON vial :

**Indication :** For severe hypoglycemic reactions in patients with D.M. treated with insulin

**Dose :** < 20 kg : 0.5 mg subcutaneous , IM or IV
> 20 kg : 1 mg subcutaneous , IM or IV

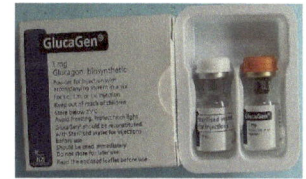

# 5- PEDIATRICS — INTRAVENOUS FLUIDS ' ESSENTIALS NOTES '..

## INTRAVENOUS FLUIDS ' ESSENTIALS NOTES ' :

### Saline :

**Note :** Isotonic , contains no glucose

**Indication :** Use for replacement of deficit in treatment of severe dehydration
As *20 cc / Kg / 1hr*   N/S ( Shoot )

**Components :** Normal saline 0.9 % ( N/S ) → $Na^+$ =150 meq/L + $Cl^-$ =150 meq/L
Ringer's lactate ( R/L ) → $Na^+$ =130 meq/L + $Cl^-$ =110 meq/L
$K^+$ =5 meq/L  + $Ca^{++}$ =2 meq/L

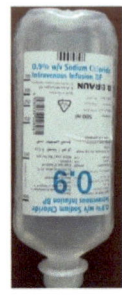 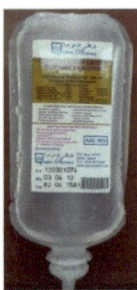

### Glucose water ( G/W ):

**Indication :** For treatment of hypoglycemic state such in
diabetic hypoglycemia
in liver disease

**Different concentrations available :**
G/W 5% → 5 gm glucose / 100 cc water
G/W 10% → 10 gm glucose / 100 cc water
G/W 50% → 50 gm glucose / 100 cc water

**Note :** 1 pint of 5% G/W → is 500 cc → so, contains 25 gm glucose
1 pint of 10% G/W → is 500 cc → so, contains 50 gm glucose
1 vial of 50% G/W ( **Hypertonic** ) → is 20 cc → so, contains 10 gm glucose

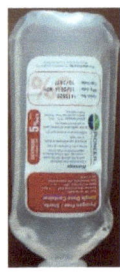 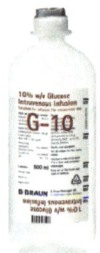 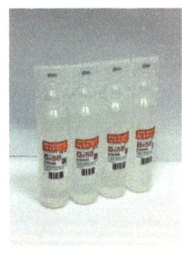

## 5- PEDIATRICS  INTRAVENOUS FLUIDS ' ESSENTIALS NOTES '..

### Glucose Saline ( G/S ):

**Indication :** For maintenance fluid requirement

**1/5 G/S Maintenance :**

$1^{st}$ 10 Kg → 100 cc / Kg
$2^{nd}$ 10 Kg → 50 cc / Kg
\> 20 Kg → 20 cc / Kg

**Components :**

1/5 Glucose Saline ( G/S ) → $Na^+$ = 30 meq/L + $Cl^-$ = 30 meq/L
Glucose = 40 gram/L

1/2 Glucose Saline ( G/S ) → $Na^+$ = 75 meq/L + $Cl^-$ = 75 meq/L
Glucose = 50 gram/L

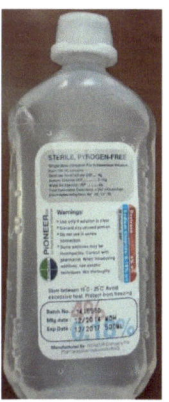

## 5- PEDIATRICS    BLOOD PRODUCTS ' ESSENTIALS NOTES '..

## Blood products ' ESSENTIALS NOTES ' :

### Whole blood :

**Indication :** Exchange transfusion

Replacement of blood loss as hypovolemia , shock , bleeding .. etc.

**Calculation :** 20 cc/kg

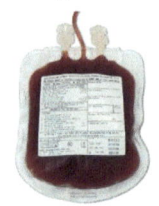

### Packed Red Blood Cells ( PRBC ) :

**Indication :** Anemia , Fluid overload , H.F. , Chronic blood loss

**Calculation :** 10 cc/kg

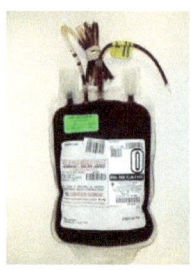

### Plasma :

**Indication :** Bleeding varices

**Calculation :** 15 cc/kg

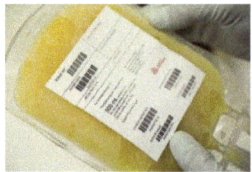

### Platelets :

**Indication :** Thrombocytopenia

**Calculation :** 1 pint / 5kg

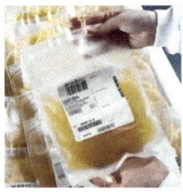

## 5- PEDIATRICS — OTHER IMPORTANT TOPICS..

### Lumbar puncture:

#### Indication:

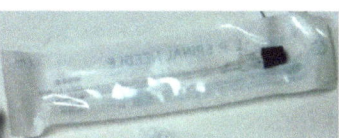

By my colleague's camera..

Diagnostic: suspected meningitis or G.B.S..
Therapeutic: drug administration,
spinal anesthesia,
decompression of spinal fluid to ↓↓ I.C.P..

#### Contraindication:

Bleeding tendency (relative), infection at the site of insertion, compromised cardiopulmonary status, & signs of ↑↑ I.C.P. in > 2 years old child (anterior fontanelle closed)..

#### Complication:

Local infection..
Trauma..
Bleeding..
Headache, backache..
Herniation..
Implantation of epidural tumor..

### Bone marrow aspiration & biopsy:

#### Indication:

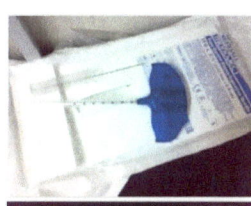

Suspicion of malignancy..
Unexplained hepatosplenomegaly..
Fever of unknown origin..
I.T.P.
Anemia of unknown cause..

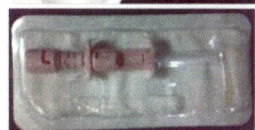

By my colleague's camera..

#### Contraindication:

Bleeding tendency..
Hypertension..
Compromises cardiopulmonary status (*unstable for G.A.*)..

#### Complication:

Local infection..
Trauma..

## 5- PEDIATRICS — OTHER IMPORTANT TOPICS..

### Exchange transfusion:

Indication:

For *indirect* hyperbilirubinemia..

The total amount of blood exchanged:

= Weight X 85 ml X 2

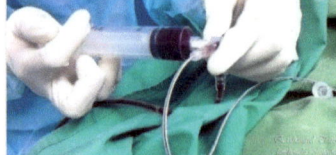

Complication:

**Acute:**

Hypoglycemia..
Hypoxia & acidosis..
Transient bradycardia with or without hypocalcaemia..
Hypocalcaemia..
Thrombosis..
Apnea with bradycardia..
Necrotizing enterocolitis (rare)..
Infection: C.M.V., H.I.V..
Death..

**Late:**

Cholestasis..
Anemia (late)..
Mild graft versus host disease..
Inspissated bile syndrome (rare)..
Portal vein thrombosis & portal hypertension..

Name of umbilical vein catheter:

Is a polyvinyl catheter..

NOTES:

- Exchange transfusion is carried out over 45 – 60 min with alternating aspiration & infusion of 20 ml of blood (each time)..
- A **calcium infusion** (1-2 ml/kg of 10% calcium gluconate given slowly via a central line) may be required to correct hypocalcaemia.

## 5- PEDIATRICS — OTHER IMPORTANT TOPICS..

### Phototherapy:

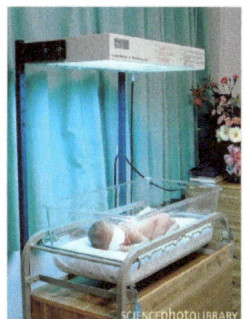

#### Indication:

For *indirect* hyperbilirubinemia..

#### Complication:

Over heating & dehydration..
Loose stool & diarrhea..
Chilling..
Eye injury & nasal closure (uncommon)..
Bronze baby syndrome..
Erythmatous maculopapular rash & purpuric rash with transient porphyria..

#### Contraindication:

Direct hyperbilirubinemia..
Porphyria..

#### NOTES:

- By using high intensity light, in the blue range 420 – 470 nm..

- The therapeutic effect of phototherapy depends on: wavelength of light, distance, amount of skin exposed & the presence of hemolysis..

- Light source distance from the infant is 45 cm, the infant should be naked except for eye patches & the baby should be turned frequently every 2 hours for maximum exposure..

- Intensive Phototherapy: used when indirect bilirubin reaches maximum level that needs exchange, so by using special light & the use of fiber optic photothearapy blanket under the baby for maximum exposure (430-490 nm wavelength)

---

### Ventolin nubulizer (Salbutamol):

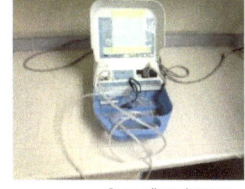

- You should educate the family about the ventolin nubulizer..
- Take 0.5 cc of ventolin then add 1.5 cc of normal saline to it..
- Put it in the nubulizer and use it over 10 – 15 minutes..
- Can repeat it 3 times only because of its side effects..

#### Indication: Asthma..

#### S.E.:

Tremor..
Tachycardia & arrhythmia..
Repeated vomiting..

## 5- PEDIATRICS    OTHER IMPORTANT TOPICS..

### Different types of drips:

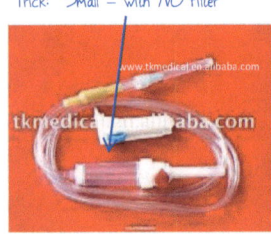
Trick: Small – with NO filter
I.V. macrodrip (15 drops = 1 ml)..

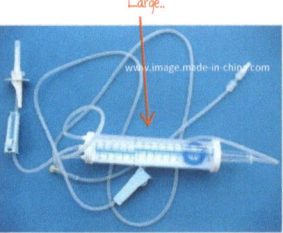
Large..
Microdrip.. (Burette-Transfusion-Set)

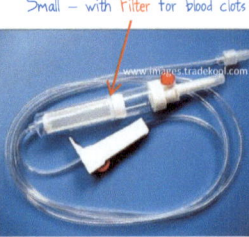
Small – with Filter for blood clots
Blood transfusion macrodrip..

#### Microdrip (Burette-Transfusion-Set):

60 drops = 1 ml

**Uses:** To give small amount of fluid..
To give some drugs (like ciprofloxacin)..
To give specific electrolytes (like $Ca^{+2}$ in 1 hour & $NaHCO_3$ in 20 min.)
*BUT NOT $K^+$..*

We close it by a simple lock to prevent any infection..

### Intraosseous needle:

#### Indication:

Difficulty in establishing venous access:
in burns, obesity, edema or seizures.
Necessity for rapid high volumes fluid infusion:
in hypovolemic shock & burns.
Access to systemic venous circulation:
in cardiopulmonary arrest, burns, medication infusion..etc

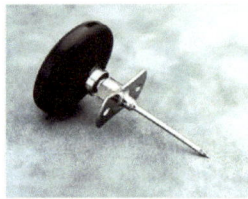

#### Contraindication:

- Infection or burn at entry site    - Osteopenia or osteopetrosis    - Osteogenesis imperfecta
- Ipsilateral fracture of extremity    - Unable to locate the landmark
- Previous attempt at the same site or diffirent location in the same bone

#### Complication:

Infection, extravasations of blood or infusion, compartment syndrome, bent needle or bone fracture ..etc

#### Positioning:

- Proximal tibia, distal to the tibial tuberosity..    - Distal end of the radial bone..
- Proximal metaphysic of the humerus..    - Distal tibia proximal to the medial malleolus..
- Distal femur, above the femur plateau..    - Sternum..    - Calcaneus..

## 5- PEDIATRICS — OTHER IMPORTANT TOPICS..

### Liver biopsy:

#### Indication:

Investigation of suspected diffuse liver disease, such as infective, autoimmune, cholestatic and congenital forms of hepatitis, metabolic liver disease, such as Wilson's disease ..etc

Investigation of focal liver disease, such as, teratoma, mesenchymal hamartoma, hepatoblastoma, rhabdoid tumour.. etc.

Management of liver transplant..

Management of drug therapies that affect the liver parenchyma..

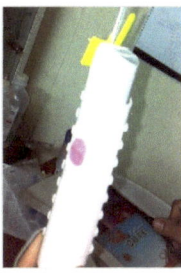

By my colleague's camera..

#### Contraindication:

A patient who is too unstable or critically unwell to undergo this procedure..

Significant coagulopathy..

Significant thrombocytopaenia..

Significant ascites..

#### Complication:

Intraperitoneal haemorrhage, biliary peritonitis, haemobilia and injury to the duodenum, colon or lung. The risk of significant bleeding after an image-guided percutaneous liver biopsy..

### Urine analysis (urine dipstick):

#### Instructions:

All samples should be midstream and collected in a clean sterile container..

Suprapubic aspiration or fresh catheter samples are ideal, but not always practical..

Immerse the dipstick completely in fresh urine and withdraw immediately, drawing edge along rim of container to remove excess..

Hold dipstick horizontally before reading..

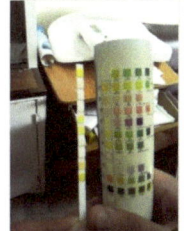

By my colleague's camera..

**For:** Color, Turbidity, Odor, Specific gravity, pH, Haematuria, Proteinuria, Glucose, Ketones, Bilirubin & Urobilinogen test, Leucocyte esterase & Urobilinogen..

### Other important topics:

#### You *have to* know something about:

- Fluid,
- Blood products,
- Drugs in pediatrics..

www.ingramcontent.com/pod-product-compliance
Lightning Source LLC
Chambersburg PA
CBHW040232220526
45473CB00001B/211